THE
CARNIVORE
DIET

Victory Belt Publishing Inc

Las Vegas

First published in 2019 by Victory Belt Publishing Inc.

Copyright © 2020 Dr. Shawn Baker

ISBN-13: 978-1-628603-50-7

The information included in this book is for educational purposes only. It is
not intended or implied to be a substitute for professional medical advice.
The reader should always consult his or her healthcare provider to determine the appropriateness of the information for his or her own situation or if
he or she has any questions regarding a medical condition or treatment plan.
Reading the information in this book does not constitute a physician-patient
relationship. The statements in this book have not been evaluated by the
Food and Drug Administration. The products or supplements in this book
are not intended to diagnose, treat, cure, or prevent any disease. The authors
and publisher expressly disclaim responsibility for any adverse effects that
may result from the use or application of the information contained in this
book.

Author photo by Jasmine Forbes
Cover design by Charisse Reyes
Interior design by Elita San Juan
Printed in Canada
TC 0119

For Jasmine, who has stood by me
through all the tough times. Thank you!

For my babies, Saxon, Emmie, Nylah, and Chouch.
Daddy loves you!

I'd like to thank the thousands of people who
have shared their life-transforming stories with
me. The driving influence behind the creation of
this book has been the phenomenal support from
the carnivore community, whose belief in actual
results over dogma has been incredibly inspiring!

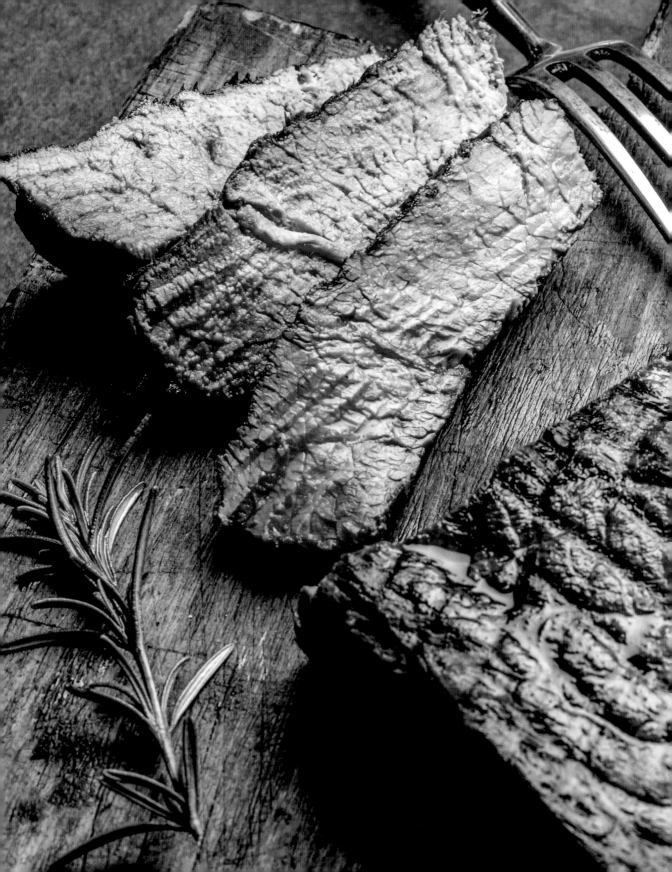

TABLE OF
CONTENTS

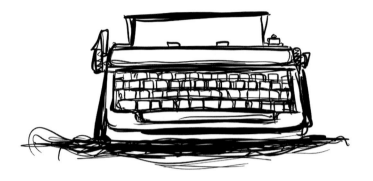

INTRODUCTION

If you would have asked me five years ago if I had plans to write a book, especially a silly diet book, I'd have said you were crazy. Well, here I am, writing a diet book and turning all the nutritional advice we've been following for at least 100 years on its ear.

This book will undoubtedly piss off a lot of people. Ethical vegans will hate it, but that's not surprising; I endorse eating meat—lots of meat. Nutritional scientists will feel threatened by it because its advice runs counter to the conventional wisdom we've been adhering to for a century, and they will decry the lack of rigorous studies on the topic. The people who will be the angriest, though, are the people who decide to adopt the carnivore diet and then find out all the stuff they've been force-fed over the years was complete garbage.

As you start to read this book, you might have doubts. The carnivore diet? What the hell? How can anyone possibly think eating a bunch of meat is anything but bad for one's health and even worse for the planet? That's certainly the message that we've heard for several generations. But here's the thing: That message has largely been unquestioned until now, and there's no real evidence to back up the claim that eating lots of meat is bad for your health.

For the last two and a half years, I've been wholly carnivorous. I haven't had a single vegetable or piece of fruit. I've had zero whole grains and not a gram of fiber. No phytonutrients or plant antioxidants have crossed my lips. Despite not eating these things, I haven't died or gotten sick. In fact, my health has been the best it's ever been. The issues that I assumed were a natural consequence of aging began to disappear. My athletic performance dramatically improved to the point that I was able to break three world records in rowing and saw my strength significantly improve.

My goal with this book is not to convince the entire world that a carnivore diet is what we all need to consume. I'm actually a bit worried that if too many people adopt this eating style, they'll cut into my supply of juicy rib-eye steaks. However, I do feel compelled to make people aware of this option and the success that many have had with this approach.

People make many assumptions about nutrition that are more firmly rooted in belief than in sound evidence. Consequently, we've seen unending attempts over the years to tailor knowledge and data to fit those deeply held beliefs. When trials produce results that run counter to those beliefs, they're dismissed and discounted. Fortunately, the times are changing, and people are starting to realize that results speak far louder than any theory. The foundations of nutrition are built on conjecture, and as more evidence comes to light, we have to work to adjust our beliefs.

Like any standard diet book in support of an argument, I refer to an assortment of scientific studies, sprinkle in some historical accounts, and get in a time machine for a bit of evolutionary guesswork. I also include some stories of life-changing experiences and personal triumphs, which I find to be at least as informative as many scientific studies. I'm not writing for the critics, of which I'm certain there will be no dearth. I'm writing for people who want to seriously change the direction of their health and life in general. Some people will get what I'm talking about, whereas others won't (or can't). I have a very difficult task ahead of me, no doubt, but I'm going to be whistling while I work and having some fun along the way!

CHAPTER **ONE** ─────────────

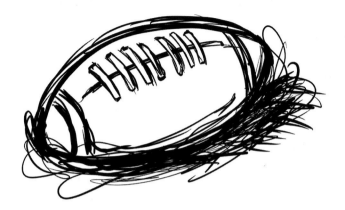

MY **STORY**

Before we get into some of the science and the rationale for the diet, it makes sense to talk about who I am, what shaped me, how I came to experiment with this diet, and why I'm now a fairly vocal advocate of it. If you don't want to read autobiographical stuff, then skip ahead to the next chapter. I promise I won't get mad.

Okay, where to start? I grew up in the 1970s, primarily living in the area near Chicago, Illinois. I became inspired to become an athlete when I saw Bruce Jenner win gold for the Olympic Decathlon in the 1976 Summer Olympics. I recall organizing my neighborhood's Olympics; winners were awarded medals that I made by wrapping stacks of pennies in aluminum foil. We included a "marathon," which was four laps around the block, sprints, a high jump into an old mattress, and a shot put event for which we used a big rock as the shot. All the kids in the neighborhood participated.

I've always been obsessed with athletics and have pushed myself to do the best I could. For some reason, I ended up fairly tall at 6′5″, even though my mother and father were only 5′1″ and 6′1″, respectively. Being tall helps for certain sports, but it limits you in others. Being a gymnast, jockey, or

CrossFit athlete would never have been in the cards for me. I was a pretty skinny guy when I was growing up. When I started high school, I was about 6'1″ and 135 pounds, which might be considered a little bit underweight. However, even at that low weight, I had a bit of a belly.

What did I eat as a kid? Pretty much the same stuff everyone else did. For breakfast I'd have sugary cereal with skim milk; Count Chocula, Fruity Pebbles, and good ol' Cap'n Crunch were my favorites. The stuff definitely tasted good, and drinking the sugar-infused milk that had turned an odd color was always the best part. Lunch was often a sandwich with some kind of lunch meat, maybe a piece of fruit, a granola bar, and perhaps some cookies. Dinner was often the standard meat, starch, and vegetables. I frequently had dessert. As I started to get older, I remember downing what must have been gallons of skim milk every week, much to the annoyance of my dad, who would come home from a long day of work to find the milk all gone. I certainly ate my share of potato chips and vanilla ice cream accompanied by chocolate cake. In fact, I sometimes would grab a can of cake frosting and just go to town with a spoon until I'd polished off the entire thing. (But don't tell my mother!)

When I was fourteen, I started to get interested in weightlifting, so I tried to make healthier food choices. I began crushing huge amounts of yogurt because I'd seen some cool television ads that implied that Russian villagers lived a long time because of yogurt. Of course, the yogurt was low fat and had tons of added sugar, but back then, the message from the experts was that we should avoid dietary fat. The sugar was less of a concern.

As I got older, I learned more information about how to get big and strong—mostly from magazines about bodybuilding. I started looking into protein powders and supplements, which I assumed were the key ingredients in making those incredibly giant, muscular guys what they were. In retrospect, it seems obvious that drug use was a huge part of bodybuilding, but at the time, I didn't know that.

By the time I was finishing high school in the great state of Texas, I had gotten up to about 195 pounds and my full adult height. According to the basketball coach, I was "the strongest kid in the school." After high school, I spent two years at a local junior college before heading off to the University of Texas in Austin to get my bachelor's degree. Around the time I turned sixteen, I had decided that I should become a doctor because I was fascinated by science and intrigued by the human body, so I studied a premed curriculum.

Of course, the yogurt was low fat and had tons of added sugar, but back then, the message from the experts was that we should avoid fat. The sugar was less of a concern.

I was busy maintaining a social life and studying while I also worked before class as a truck loader for UPS. Even with such a full calendar, I still found time to train. I discovered I had a natural talent for picking up heavy things and putting them down. My boss at UPS, Jerry, was basically about my age and went to the same gym I did. He said he would load my trucks if I could deadlift a bar loaded to 455 pounds. I was nineteen at the time, and I'd never deadlifted *any* weight, much less the 455 pounds in the challenge. I approached the bar, grabbed it, and pulled for all I was worth. To the surprise of both Jerry and me, the bar came off the floor, and I locked it out. Lifting that 455 pounds set me on a path of a lifelong love affair with the deadlift. In the year 2000, I eventually pulled 772 pounds and set a drug-free American powerlifting record. (By the way, that SOB Jerry never did load those trucks for me.)

I transferred to the University of Texas, where I continued to train hard and study hard. I earned my biology degree and was accepted to medical school.

I Begin My Medical Career and Take a Detour

I started medical school at the University of Texas Medical Branch at Galveston, Texas. Shortly after arriving in Galveston, I found a great gym—Sergeant Rock's Gym—that was owned by a cat named Paul McCartney (no, not the Beatle). Paul jokingly stated that if I wished to continue to train at his gym, then I had to play for the local rugby team. Becoming a rugby player turned out to be a life-altering event for me on several levels.

I had never even watched rugby, but I naturally took to it because I was athletic, big, strong, and fast. After an initial introduction, I was hooked. Soon my main interest was in training for rugby, and the medical school stuff became a secondary priority. I was still getting decent grades, but I wasn't performing at the level I could have if school had been my main focus. As I got more proficient at rugby, I began to make some all-star and select side teams. Soon I was traveling all over the country playing for the All-Texas team and then later for the Western U.S. team.

Due to my travels for rugby, I ended up missing one of the labs for my pharmacology class. I had the opportunity to make up the lab, but I did the math to figure out how it would affect my grade and realized I could still easily get an A in the class, even with a zero score on that particular lab. So I told the pharmacology department's secretary that I was okay with skipping it. Apparently, that didn't go over too well, and I quickly found myself on academic probation. Around the time this occurred, I received an offer to go to New Zealand, the rugby Mecca of the world, to play for one of the premiere-level club teams. After about five minutes of intense deliberation, I said, "Hell, yeah! Screw this medical school stuff. I'm heading to Kiwi-land." I withdrew from medical school, much to the shock of my professors, and headed to New Zealand.

Rugby is not a sport for the meek. It can be savage, but it's also beautifully artistic when it's executed with skill. I thoroughly enjoyed my time in New Zealand and do not regret for one second my decision to drop out of medical school to go there. While I was in New Zealand, I had all sorts of odd jobs, including garbage man, gas line digger, sheep shearer, dairy deliverer, and bartender. As the "imported American," I was often invited to people's homes for dinner, which almost invariably was some sort of lamb dish served with a roasted kumara, which is basically the Kiwi version of a sweet potato. I ate so much lamb while I was there that a decade passed before I wanted to eat it again. (Ironically, as the carnivore diet eater I am now, I eat beef every single day, and I've never lost the taste for it. I also thoroughly enjoy lamb when I can get it.)

When I finished my stint in New Zealand, I headed back to Texas. I needed a job, and at that time, the military had one of the best rugby programs in the country, so I joined the United States Air Force. I went to Officer Training School, where I excelled and graduated with distinction. I earned a regular commission, which is a fairly rare event for people who aren't Air Force Academy graduates. I was too tall to be a pilot, though, and I didn't have perfect vision, so I was sent off to learn how to launch nuclear warheads attached to intercontinental ballistic missiles. I had to pass a battery of personality and psychological reliability tests before I was accepted and given my top secret security clearance.

After about six months in California at Vandenberg Air Force Base, learning all the intricacies of the Minuteman III Nuclear weapons control system, I was packed up and sent up to F. E. Warren Air Force Base in Cheyenne, Wyoming. For five years, I worked twenty-four-hour shifts up to eight times a month to babysit as many as 150 nuclear warheads and practice regularly for World War III. I was pretty decent at pretending to launch nuclear bombs and was named Missile Combat Crew Commander of the year. Eventually, I became an instructor.

As I finished out my twenties, playing rugby became less interesting to me. During one match against a team from Russia, one of the Russian athletes repeatedly kicked me in the head. Blood was pouring from one of my ears, and I decided that it was time for me to hang up the cleats and look into getting a "real career." Surprisingly, there wasn't a great deal

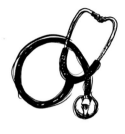

of demand for nuclear weapons launch officers in the civilian sector. Fortunately, I was able to talk the military into paying for me to go back to medical school.

First, I had to be reaccepted to medical school. Unfortunately, this is where my past came back to bite me in the ass. Because my GPA during my last semester of college had been low, I needed to take a ton of college courses to bring up my average. I enrolled in distance learning at the University of Wyoming and began knocking out classes at a furious pace, getting nothing but straight As, so I was able to bring my overall college GPA back into the "med-school-acceptable range." I also had to retake the MCAT, which is the standardized test for people who want to go to medical school. Fortunately, I basically aced that test, which made me a fairly strong candidate to get back into school. I ended up getting into Texas Tech University.

Once I was back in medical school, I was determined to kick ass. At that point, I weighed about 285 to 300 pounds and was very good at setting powerlifting records, but I wasn't great at staying awake in class. When I look back on that time and consider what I've learned about nutrition since then, I strongly suspect a typical garbage high-carbohydrate diet was largely responsible for my somnolence.

I studied the textbooks thoroughly, though, and I routinely received among the highest scores on the tests, which is crucial if you want to succeed and have your choice of specialties. You also have to kick ass during the clinical rotations. You have to hustle and get your work done. Being an athlete gave me a physical leg up on the competition because I could work like a dog without wearing out. My eye was on the prize, and that prize was a residency in orthopedic surgery. At the end of my four years in medical school, I graduated near the top of the class and secured my first choice of orthopedic surgical residency programs, which was back at the University of Texas—the very same place from which I had dropped out of medical school nearly a decade prior.

I started my surgical residency at the Shriner Hospitals for Children pediatric burn care center, which is one of the largest and most well-known burn hospitals in the United States. It was largely a horrifying experience! I was completely clueless, exhausted, and questioning what I was doing and why I wanted to be a surgeon. I was on call every third night, which meant that I was responsible for an entire intensive care unit of sick, horribly burned kids, many of whom were close to death. Thanks to the support of the veteran nurses who had been working in this area for years, I managed to get through it even though I was a naïve, inexperienced doctor. After that initial trial by fire, I spent the rest of my intern year rotating through the various surgical subspecialties.

After four years of medical school and five long years of residency, my training was finally over, or at least I thought it was. I had graduated my residency with numerous awards and received the sign-off I needed to be released on my own into the wild.

I would be remiss if I didn't mention that my first child was born just as I was finishing my residency. Saxon Michael Baker arrived into the world in the early morning hours of March 26, 2006. He was a strikingly beautiful little boy, and his presence changed my life forever! It wasn't until he was about 18 months old that we started to figure out that he was not quite the same as other children. By age three, he officially was diagnosed with autism. Later, two wonderful little girls, Emmie and Nylah, joined my family; eventually, my fourth child, Lucas, was born.

Because Uncle Sam had paid for my medical school tuition, the government wanted its pound of flesh once I was fully trained. In the early part of 2006, I reentered the Air Force with the rank of major and began to practice routine stateside orthopedics. My first "solo" surgery was a knee scope—something I had done hundreds of times in my residency, and it went well. Once I had that first surgery under my belt, things started to fall into a regular pattern, and the job was largely very enjoyable. Unfortunately, the easy life of taking care of mostly healthy and young active military personnel and their families came to an abrupt halt in January 2007, when I was sent to Afghanistan for six months to take care of the war casualties.

War Zone

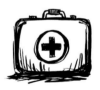

They say, "War is hell," and I gotta tell you, they're right. During my surgical residency, I had taken care of train crash victims and the casualties from a refinery explosion. Those accidents pale in comparison to the amount of human devastation that we unleash upon each other while at war. There was not a single day during my time in Afghanistan that we were not inundated with horrific casualties. We operated nonstop every day, all day long, taking breaks only to eat, get a little exercise, and sleep when there was a lull in the action at night.

When I went to the Middle East, I was just six months from graduating from my surgical residency, and I was thrust into one of the worst combat places on Earth. My fantastic orthopedic colleague, Dr. Tom Large (who also was fresh out of residency), and I were the orthopedic trauma specialists for the *entire* Afghanistan war zone. We saw everything: fresh trauma from the local area, day-old trauma that had been hastily bundled up from the forward operating bases, kids, adults, U.S. soldiers, NATO forces, Afghan Army, good guys, bad guys, prisoners of war, Taliban soldiers, and high-level operatives. When we had time, we even did some mission work for local adults and kids who had joint deformities or other chronic orthopedic issues. I have never been, nor will I ever again be, as busy as I was during that time. I'd like to think that I came out of my frontline military experience without any mental scars, but I've noticed that it's now viscerally painful for me to see people getting injured in movies or TV shows, which is something that never used to bother me.

At the end of my deployment, some two-star general, whom I had never seen before and whose name I can't remember, pinned a medal on my chest. I was relieved to be going home and glad as hell to be out of that place. One of the other surgeons summed it up like this: "It was a million-dollar experience that I would not have paid a nickel for." I can honestly say that after that experience, there was nothing I could ever see that would bother me. War is still hell, but if I have one good thing to say about it, it's that it teaches us a lot about medicine—and, honestly, about life in general.

When I got home, my son Saxon had grown from a little baby into a small boy who cried when he saw me coming off the plane. It took me several months to acclimate to life back at home, but eventually, things began to normalize. I was named the chief of orthopedics at the Air Force base where I was stationed, and then I transferred to another base where I was also named the chief of orthopedics. When my five years with the Air Force were up, I decided to get out of the military and enter civilian practice. I separated with the rank of lieutenant colonel.

Civilian Clothes

Transitioning from military life to civilian practice was actually fairly easy. I had been separated from my family for about two years, and it was nice to be with them regularly. I joined a small, fairly low-speed orthopedic group of just two other doctors. After an initial welcome period, the administration asked me to lead the group. I accepted that responsibility and quickly helped grow the group from three relatively low-productivity surgeons into a larger group of twelve providers in two locations. We had the dominant business on our side of town, and we were thriving.

In addition to my duties as the head of the group, I had an incredibly busy clinical schedule. I routinely saw forty to fifty patients a day, and I supervised several physician's assistants and nurse practitioners. My operating room schedule was packed, and I often did close to 600 surgeries a year, which is roughly double the national average for a general orthopedist. I was busy, but my patients were generally happy, the results were good, and the hospital was pleased with the revenue from my work and the work of the group.

Dark Days and a Change in Diet

Unfortunately, not everything was perfect. In 2012, I went through a divorce and lost daily contact with my kids. This was one of the most painful experiences I had ever dealt with; it's still painful to this day. I suffered in silence and let only a few of my closest friends at work know what was going on. I kept up my grueling work schedule and started to medicate myself with intense exercise.

After a long period, I found myself in a new relationship with a wonderful and incredibly supportive woman, Jasmine, who helped get me back on my feet. She's still hanging strong with me today. (Interestingly, when I met Jasmine, she was largely vegetarian, which I found particularly odd because she hails from France—the land of Chateaubriand, butter, and cream.)

The silver lining behind my troubles is that I began to take notice of my health. I was approaching my mid-forties, but I was still training like a beast. In fact, I had recently been crowned a Highland Games Masters World Champion. Despite my considerable strength and my efforts at training, in retrospect, I can see that I was developing metabolic syndrome. By no means would the average person have concluded that I was fat. I was a big guy, about 280 pounds, but the weight was mostly muscle—at least that's what I told myself. I wasn't sleeping well, I snored a lot, I was often tired, and I clearly had sleep apnea. My blood pressure was starting to creep up, and as time went on, I experienced more and more aches and pains. As a successful athlete and surgeon, I had a hard time accepting that I was becoming unhealthy. My dietary philosophy of "eat what you want as long as you train hard enough" had caught up with me. Mind you, I never ate copious amounts of junk food, but I could binge on ice cream, pizza, or other hyperpalatable foods from time to time. I ate plenty of fruit, lots of lean dairy (I was still pounding down the yogurt), and lots of cereals and pasta to get in my whole grains. I loved meat, and I wasn't much of a vegetable fan. I ate *a lot* of food.

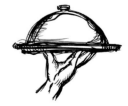

Once I realized that I could no longer rely only on exercise to keep me healthy, I decided to make a dietary change. My knowledge of nutrition up to that point consisted of what most physicians know, plus a little bit of stuff I'd read to help me as an athlete. My first step was to reduce the calories I consumed; I went from eating about 6,000 calories per day to about 3,000. I cut out junk food and sugar, and I started eating plenty of leafy green vegetables, lots of fibrous foods, and just a small amount of lean meat like chicken and fish. I ramped up my exercise and started jumping rope—1,000 skips first thing in the morning. At lunch, I did a weight workout. When I got home in the evening, I did another 1,000 jump rope skips. Weight quickly started to fly off—within the first month I dropped 30 pounds. I further reduced my calories and upped my jump rope routine to 2,000 and then 3,000 skips per session. Over the next two months, I was down an additional 20 pounds for a total of 50 pounds in three months. I was lean, and I looked much better (even though the nurses said I was getting too skinny). I also was constantly starving, and I was miserable.

At this point, I started looking into Paleo-style diets and experimenting with altering my eating habits according to those guidelines. I felt better. My weight remained fairly stable, and I started learning to cook Paleo recipes. I read several books on nutrition and became immersed in popular books on the subject. At some point, I read *Good Calories, Bad Calories* by Gary Taubes and was blown away by the flaws in our understanding of nutrition. Taubes's book caused me to question much of the dogma that I had previously accepted without a second thought. I later read Nina Teicholz's book *The Big Fat Surprise* and was equally impressed by the corruption that influenced what we were being advised to eat. I went further down the low-carb rabbit hole and read books by Stephen Phinney, Jeff Volek, Jimmy Moore, and Jason Fung. Eventually, I ended up following a ketogenic-style diet, and for the first time, I knew what it was like to be free of hunger.

I went all in on keto, buying recipe books and making all kinds of foods, including delicious desserts. I was adding MCT oil to my food in the hope that I was upping my ketone levels. To improve my athletic performance, I starting playing with both the targeted and cyclic versions of the ketogenic diet. On some of the carb-up days, I really struggled to choke down all the carbs I had calculated that I should consume. At first, I looked forward to the carb refeeds. As time went on, though, I noticed that not only did I not enjoy them, but my gastrointestinal tract didn't like them, and my performance in the gym was not discernibly better.

Ultimately, I was very much a ketogenic diet advocate. I included meat in my diet, and I often took my entire office to eat prime rib at the local barbecue place when it was the Friday special. I ate plenty of bacon and eggs, but at the same time, I was eating massive spinach salads topped with olive oil, nuts, eggs, bacon, and a few berries.

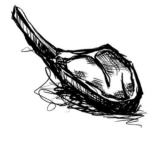

As my health continued to improve, I started to talk to some of my obese patients about the ketogenic diet. I was excited to share a tool that I felt would work for them. I printed flyers with reading assignments and recommended videos that explained some of the science behind the diet and how to implement it. For a high percentage of the patients to whom I recommended the ketogenic diet, it worked.

Soon I started seeing that many of the orthopedic conditions I commonly had treated with drugs, injections, or surgery started to resolve with just the diet. I dug through the literature to find out what was going on. Unfortunately, not much data existed about the relationship between diet and common orthopedic conditions. I found a handful of studies that examined clinical conditions that generally supported what I was observing in my patients, and I also found a fair bit of basic science research that supported my growing hypothesis. With the continued success that I was seeing, I became more excited. I was giving flyers to just about every patient who expressed even the slightest bit of interest.

I couldn't contain my enthusiasm about the results of the diet. Even though I loved being in the operating room, I was more invested in seeing my patients get better in every aspect of their health as they changed what they ate. Instead of feeling like a cog in the wheel, I felt empowered. I was attaining what I always had hoped for when I dreamed about being a doctor when I was a sixteen-year-old kid.

I met with my chief administrator to talk about the results I was seeing in my patients, and he politely told me that it was interesting, but he didn't share my enthusiasm. I began to hint that I would like to have some dedicated clinic time to practice a lifestyle medicine approach. My hints were largely ignored. I thought that this dietary approach might apply to the employee wellness program, so I scheduled a meeting with the head of the program. When I got to her office and saw a giant container of peaches on her desk, though, I realized that she was all in on the "plant-based" diet. I effectively got nowhere with her.

The hospital had just hired a full-time bariatric surgeon who was someone I got along with very well. Part of the bariatric program was supposed to include a nonoperative diet-based practice. That part never got off the ground, although the surgical part was chugging along nicely. I asked if I could run the dietary portion part-time; the response was basically "No thanks." Finally, in frustration, I started changing my schedule. Instead of the usual eight-minute visits, I was spending forty minutes in the room with my patients. Instead of booking loads of surgeries every day, I began to suggest that perhaps we should hold off on surgery and try diet and other lifestyle modifications. My nurse was constantly printing new flyers because I went through an entire stack every few days. The hospital administrators told me that there wasn't much appetite for all this lifestyle stuff in the orthopedic department. But, as the head of the group, I didn't much care what the administrators thought, and I continued to move forward.

Eventually, I had to meet with someone from medical staff affairs, and that person informed me that policies had recently changed. During an audit of my office records from several years prior, the auditor had discovered that I fell into the category that could warrant a peer-review process. I was told that a dozen random cases would be selected and reviewed by another orthopedic surgeon.

A few months later, I was called back into the office and told that the review of my cases had been completed, and several of them were deemed "below average." I asked to look at the cases but was told that I wasn't allowed to see them. (I later found out that policy was inaccurate; I should have been allowed to provide clarification about the cases that had been reviewed.) I also found out that the reviewer of my cases just happened to have been employed by the crosstown rival group to my practice. I expressed my concern that a direct financial competitor was being allowed to review my cases. The administrators agreed that a possible conflict of interest could exist and that they would send my cases to an independent outside review company. I was told that most of the issues identified were about how I documented my records, and I was reassured that I likely had nothing to worry about. I went back to work taking care of patients.

Another few months passed, and I received a message from the administrator that I was to cancel my next day's clinic and any upcoming operations; I was to meet with the administrator that afternoon. When I arrived, the administrator gave me a copy of the outside reviewer's report, which contained a brief identification of the cases that had been chosen without any further identifying information or details. The report listed several deficiencies in my care and stated that on numerous occasions, I had performed a surgery that was not indicated, was poorly documented, or was otherwise problematic. As I read the report, my heart sank, and I fell into a state of shock. I was informed that effective immediately, my hospital privileges were provisionally suspended pending formal review by a committee.

As you might imagine, this type of review is incredibly stressful and emotionally taxing. The next day, the president of the hospital staff, who would sit on the committee to determine my fate, asked if I wanted to meet for breakfast and talk about any concerns I might have. He told me that based on that outside review report, it was almost guaranteed that I would be formally suspended, and he suggested that I write a letter to the committee and basically "fall on my sword" in the hope of a better outcome. Still numb and in shock, I agreed to write the letter and did as he suggested, thinking that he had my best interest in mind.

Depressed as hell, I drove out to the Grand Canyon to meet up with my girlfriend. I spent the next few days in a zombielike state while I waited for the committee to meet. As expected, the committee delivered the suspension verdict. I was told that it was a very difficult decision because all the members who knew who I was and had worked with me had always found me very likable; they'd never observed any problems with my patient care. However, the committee comprised physicians from various nonorthopedic specialties, and they deferred to the information in the report. An orthopedic advisor was available to the committee by conference call, but I learned that the advisor was another member of the crosstown rival practice.

At first, I accepted my fate and told the hospital that I wouldn't contest the findings. I spent the next few weeks sitting at home trying to figure out what the heck I was going to do with my life. As my state of shock wore off, though, I started to get angry. I consulted with a lawyer, and I submitted a request for a fair hearing to proceed without the influence of any direct financial competitors.

My lawyer asked that we be allowed access to all the records that had been part of the review on which the suspension decision was based. When I was able to review those records and the report, I was shocked because I could see that the independent reviewer had made numerous blatant errors and clearly had been influenced by the original report from my crosstown rival; the report wasn't an independent review. I was very upset, of course, but at least I was allowed to point out where multiple errors had been made in the report.

When the day of my hearing finally arrived, I listened silently as the hospital presented its case, which downplayed the fact that the outside review was the crucial piece of evidence that ultimately caused the committee to suspend me. The hospital claimed that I had once used the word *bullshit* in an email, and the administrators were going to suspend me regardless of the outside report. This assertion was in complete contrast to what I had been told all along. It seemed that the hospital knew that the report was a piece of garbage and was trying to pretend it was only of minimal relevance. I was very frustrated by the testimony.

When it was my turn to make my case, my attorney and I destroyed the integrity of the outside reviewer's report. At the end of the hearing, I was told that the hearing officer would generate a report by the end of the month. For the rest of that month, I anxiously checked the mail every day; when the results finally arrived, I tore into the envelope and began to read. The results conceded that the report from the independent reviewer was bogus and full of problems. However, the hearing officer, whom we had objected to because he had recently retired from the employment of my direct financial competitor, stated that it was clear that I had been giving my patients "too much choice" when it came to determining their treatment options. He concluded that the hospital was right to suspend me. I am still

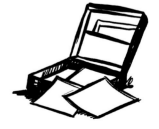

flabbergasted at the concept of giving a patient "too much choice" when it comes to their medical care!

Needless to say, I was disappointed with that outcome. A short time afterward, the state medical board got involved because the hospital had filed a formal complaint. I had two options. The first was to challenge the complaint and have a state-level hearing; however, a year or more could pass before the date of the hearing, and mounting my defense would likely be very expensive. I'd already gone nearly two years without being able to earn any income, and my savings had dwindled. I knew the hospital would continue to invest in their interest over the truth. So I chose the second option, which was to be evaluated completely independently if I voluntarily surrendered my medical license.

I went to Denver, Colorado, where an independent agency spent several days evaluating me as I worked through a series of physical, mental, and neurocognitive tests, interviews with several orthopedic surgeons, simulated patient encounters, and a review of my patient charts. At the end of the evaluation, I was told that the agency would prepare a report with the results of the evaluation. Four months later, I received the report, which stated that I was completely competent to return to practice as soon as possible. I was instructed to update some continuing medical education because I had been out of practice for well over two years. Of course, I was happy with those results and felt somewhat vindicated. My license was reinstated after more than three and a half years of waiting.

I Go Off the Deep End and Become a True Meathead

While all the controversy about my medical practice was happening, I continued to devour writings and scientific literature on nutrition and lifestyle. I continued to experiment with my nutrition and other lifestyle practices. In early 2016, I started to get interested in a group of people who appeared to be thriving by eating a pure carnivore diet. I had seen improvements in some areas while following a ketogenic-style diet, but people who were following this crazy all-meat diet were reporting even more improvements with far more frequency and success. How could it be that people who had already been eating a low-carb or ketogenic diet and had already cut out sugars, seed oils, and refined grains could be getting healthier by giving up spinach, broccoli, and kale? It did not compute. Everything I had ever read or heard before was that these foods were the keys to health, and no one questioned the truth of that wisdom. Sure, I had heard of societies (like the Inuit and Maasai) who lived primarily on meat, but these people did those things because of their unusual living conditions. Of course, I knew that those cultures were noted to be exceptionally healthy, but I had assumed that their good health was due to the lack of junk food and the inclusion of lots of physical activity.

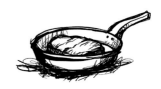

As I became more and more fascinated by this crazy phenomenon of people thriving by eating only meat, I began to look more deeply into the available literature. I read the writings of Vilhjalmur Stefansson, who described how he spent more than a decade living among the Inuit and eating an exclusively meat-based diet. He claimed that he never felt better than he did during that period. I looked through numerous peer-reviewed studies that occurred after Stefansson agreed to eat only meat for one year to prove to the skeptical scientific world that it could be done. I saw the conclusions that stated that he and his partner in the study were in excellent health after the one-year trial; they were free from any deficiencies or illness.

I recognized an amazing simplicity in the diet and could see how intuitively easy it was. I saw a growing community that was tired of the complexity, the frustration, and the futility that were so common with other nutritional advice. This idea of a meat-only diet was about eating for the sake of nutrition without regard for social pressures, entertainment aspects, addictions, or expectations. Sure, some people who tried it struggled to adapt, but many were getting healthy and were redefining their relationship with food. Eating became easy, and anxieties began to disappear. For the first time in their lives, people were experiencing true nutritional satisfaction, and it was infectious. I wanted to try it. I had always loved the taste of meat, but in the back of my mind, I'd always felt a slight sense of guilt—not because I was eating an animal but because I had been told that eating a lot of meat and not eating copious amounts of fruits and vegetables was bad for me.

Throughout the summer of 2016, I started having carnivore days. I would eat eggs, bacon, seafood, steaks, and hamburgers. I enjoyed the heck out of it; honestly, I felt pretty darn good. On some days, I would eat more "normal" foods, and on those days I didn't feel as well. I began to look forward to my carnivore days. Slowly I went from having a few carnivore days at a time to a week at a time. Surprisingly, I didn't miss eating other foods. Then one week became ten days, and then it stretched to two weeks. The whole time I was feeling great.

Toward the end of 2016, I had become fairly active on social media, particularly Twitter, and I announced to my followers that I would be doing a crazy thirty-day carnivore challenge. Lots of humorous posts followed that announcement, and I even ran a poll to let people predict what I would die of. Was I going to get scurvy? Would my arteries immediately clog up? Would my colon fall out? A few people took the carnivore challenge with me and had a good time sharing their results. At the end of the month, I had survived, and I hadn't developed scurvy or any other malady. Other than having a mild headache for the first week or so, the month had gone very well, and I'd quite enjoyed it.

The day after the thirty-day challenge ended, I ate the foods that I thought I had been missing. I had some fruit, some nuts, and a couple of other things, and I observed that my previously perfect digestion was somewhat uncomfortable. I noticed a return of a slight bit of back pain, and I didn't feel particularly satisfied when I ate. My original intention was to limit my experiment to just thirty days, but I discovered that I much preferred the way I felt on the all-meat diet. The next day, I went right back on the diet and continued to talk about it on social media. Even though I continued to get healthier every week and started to see my strength and athletic performance skyrocket, many people said I was doing myself harm. Not long after, I began to attract the attention of a horde of online critics who were vegans.

At first, I engaged these folks and tried to have an intelligent discussion. Soon I realized that these people were completely invested in an ideology and would not be swayed no matter what facts were presented to them. I quickly found that when I asked, "Would you eat meat if it would improve your health?" the answer was always, "No!" To me, this response indicated complete irrationality; I muted and eventually blocked these people on social media because interacting with them became a huge waste of time and energy. Ironically, some of them ultimately told me that they gave up veganism and improved their health after following my work.

My two months on the meat-only diet turned into six months, and still I was being criticized for my experiment; critics said that my results were in no way reflective of what most people should expect. At this point, I decided that it might be interesting to see if my results truly were isolated or if other people could expect the same. I conducted another online poll to see if anyone would be interested in eating a bunch of steaks for ninety days. Within a few days, I had hundreds of volunteers. At that point, Matt Maier, another carnivore and Air Force veteran, and I decided to organize a "study," even though we had no funding or any other support. The "research team" was the two of us doing what we could in our spare time. I created a web page called Nequalsmany.com, and we collected names of volunteers.

By August 2016, several hundred people had signed up to participate, and off they went, tearing through steaks and burgers, giving up coffee and carbs. At the end of the ninety days, we had lots of data. It took us something like six months to analyze and sort it all. No participants got scurvy, and no one died or had any significant problems. The vast majority of people lost significant weight and belly fat. Most were eating at least two pounds of meat per day, and subjectively almost all participants saw significant improvements (indigestion, joint health, and sleep habits). Admittedly, this little "scientific experiment" had issues that could lead critics to be dismissive of the results. For example, the study had a selection and a survivor bias, there was no control group, and we didn't control what people ate. Many of the outcomes were subjective, and several confounders (such as exercise) could have influenced the outcome. The upshot of the trial, however, is that a bunch of people ate a meat-based diet, and the vast majority of them got healthier.

More and more people started to take notice of my work, and soon I was being asked to be a guest on podcasts and in other interviews. Joe Rogan, who arguably has one of the most influential podcasts in the world, invited me on his show. As a result, millions of people became exposed to the carnivore diet. Most saw it as crazy—including Joe, in all likelihood. More and more vegans started attacking me; some even compared me to Satan and Hitler. Despite the criticism, interest in my crazy diet preference took off. I tried to accommodate as many interviews as I could and tried to present a fair and nondogmatic approach to the diet. In the mainstream media, I often was portrayed as a bit crazy, if not dangerous. Most of the articles that included my story started with, "Dr. Shawn Baker, who had his medical license revoked, blah, blah, blah." The pushback against the diet is extreme, to say the least.

Registered dietitians are regularly trotted out by the media to warn you of the dangers of attempting a meat-based diet. The claim is that the diet is so preposterous that even attempting it will result in a health crisis. The dietitians say that if it doesn't kill you immediately, you surely are condemning yourself to a future of cardiovascular disease, colon cancer, and diabetes. They pay no attention to the results showing that essentially every risk factor for those issues tends to go away when a person follows the diet, and they ignore the fact that societies that eat meat-based diets are free of those diseases. Many of those cultures don't even have words for the conditions. People who follow the diet—like Mikhaila Peterson, daughter of controversial Canadian psychologist Jordan Peterson—were accused of lying about their medical conditions, and critics claimed that the only reason people were getting healthy was that they'd lost some weight. Long-term carnivores (people who've followed

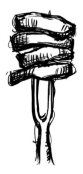

the diet for ten years or more)—like Joe and Charlene Andersen and Charles Washington—were accused of keeping themselves alive by secretly eating fruit and other foods. Surely eating meat alone can't be good for us; that would be too much of a challenge to our nutritional beliefs. Even though humans have been eating meat since humans have existed, people now want to blame it for our modern epidemic of disease.

As one year on the carnivore diet turned into two, I saw continued improvements in my health, body composition, and athletic performance, and thousands of other people noticed similar changes in themselves. Every single day I received letters of encouragement that included amazing stories about how people's lives had been changed by eating this way. People lost weight, reduced or eliminated medications, and started to participate in life again. Depression that had lasted decades faded, and chronic pain disappeared. I was so moved that I started another website called Meatheals.com with carnivore Michael Goldstein. We began collecting and organizing these incredible anecdotes and sorted them by condition for easy reference. We still receive daily submissions.

As the media continued to struggle with the carnivore diet, many people tried to politicize it by claiming it was a diet of right-wing conservatives and neo-Nazis. Sometimes during interviews, I could sense the reporters trying to steer me into confirming their suspicions that I was involved in a right-wing conspiracy, like they thought I'd say that anyone who eats only meat must somehow harbor anti-gay, racist, or other bigoted tendencies. For the record, I am none of those things, and I have seen people of all races, religions, sexual orientations, and political leanings adopt this diet with success. A delicious steak does not care who you voted for!

I hope you enjoyed hearing a bit about my story. We all have to write our own stories, and yours might be very different from mine. No one can decide what is right for you; you must come to that decision on your own. My only recommendation is for you objectively to assess what is important to you. Base your decisions on your needs rather than what your family, friends, doctor, or society as a whole wants for you. You're the one who has to walk around and sleep in the only body you will ever own. How you choose to live and take care of that body is up to you. Can the carnivore diet serve some purpose for you? I can't say for certain, but the rest of this book might help answer some of your questions.

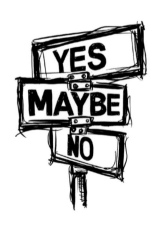

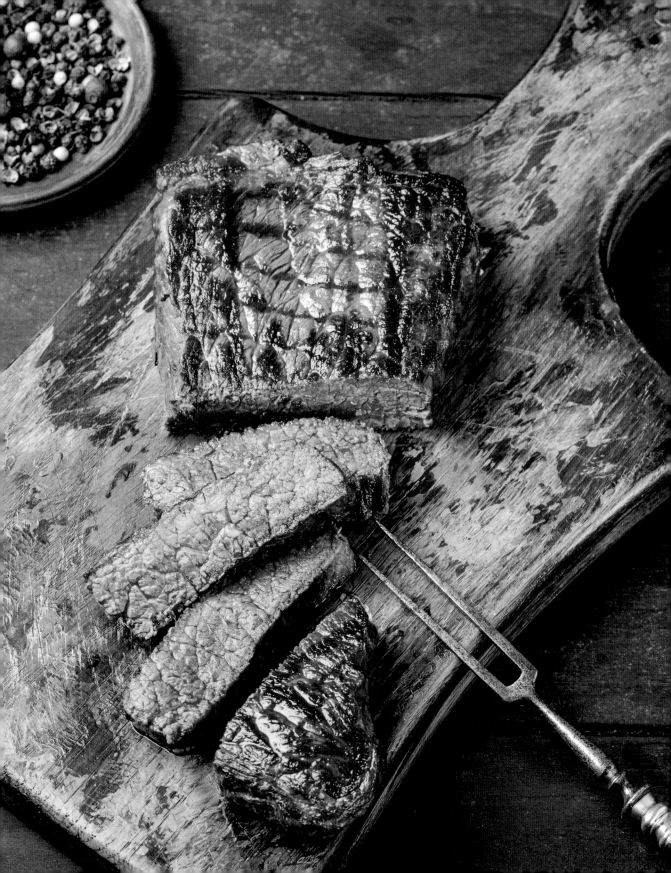

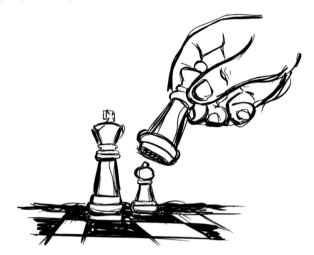

CHAPTER TWO

WHERE DID WE
GO WRONG?

"The biggest problem is that the vast majority of studies are not experimental, randomized designs. Simply by observing what people eat—or even worse, what they recall they ate—and trying to link this to disease outcomes is moreover a waste of effort. These studies need to be largely abandoned. We've wasted enough resources and caused enough confusion."

—Professor John Ioannidis, MD, 2018

I'm going to be blunt: Much of human nutritional research has been a heaping pile of garbage on which we've wasted gazillions of dollars. The result is that everyone is fat, sick, weak, tired, and depressed, or they're running around with calculators to track every morsel of food they eat. That's the politest way I can describe it. More people probably have been killed, injured, or psychologically damaged because of stupid nutritional advice than in the combination of all the wars that have happened in the last century.

One of the oft-heard refrains from the research intelligentsia is that it's very difficult (even nearly impossible) to do truly meaningful nutrition research on humans. That's true. To thoroughly test which diet is best, you would need to lock multiple pairs of twins in a metabolic ward for their entire lives and control for every single variable to ensure they eat the exact diets you are testing. Experiments such as those would be unethical, and they'll never be done.

Instead, we often do large-scale population studies in which we ask people to guesstimate what they've eaten over the previous six months. Then we try our best to control for the thousands of different lifestyle confounders. How much someone drinks, smokes, wears a seatbelt, visits the doctor, exercises, spends time outdoors, meditates, or sleeps can affect that person's health. We can only guess what effects these types of confounders will have, especially as they vary from person to person. We can do animal studies, often using mice or rats; unfortunately, very often, those results are impossible to extrapolate to humans.

Another alternative is to do short-term interventions and look at some proxy lab marker that we think may be (kind of, sort of) linked to some disease in some cases. As uncertain as animal and short-term intervention studies are, we have to make do with the information we can glean from them. It's a bit like saying, "The airplane you're about to board has only one wing, and the engine seems to be failing, but that's the best we have. Good luck!" I don't know about you, but I ain't too keen on flying on that plane.

Nutrition Is Complicated

We seem to learn new stuff every week about how complicated human metabolism is. Each time someone makes a discovery, we speculate about what it might mean. Supplement companies rush to market with the latest product that goes with the new knowledge. People buy up the supplements and wonder if they're having any effect. A few years go by; no one uses the supplements anymore, but guess what? Someone makes another discovery, and the cycle repeats ad infinitum.

Today we walk around with devices that tell us exactly how many steps we've taken and measure all kinds of variables, including heart rate, sleep patterns, and blood glucose. We spend hours obsessing over macro- and micronutrients. We calculate our eating windows to the nearest minute. We're knowledge-empowered and optimized, and, for a brief period, we think we have a solution. "It's all about calories," cries one camp. "It's all about carbs and insulin," declares another. "You just need the perfect amount of balance and moderation" is the mantra from a third camp. Meanwhile, every other animal on the planet is just hanging out, munching on grass or chewing zebra bones or whatever. Strangely, those other species aren't suffering and getting fat because they can't use all these high-tech tools and data. (Last year, I gave my dog a FitBit for his birthday, but he just chewed on it for a while and then stopped playing with it. I guess he wasn't smart enough to figure it out.)

What if, by some crazy, lucky coincidence, human beings were also animals, and there exists a diet they could eat that doesn't involve obsessive planning, calculating, and tracking? What if you could just eat when you feel hungry? What if you could get what you need to stay healthy from the food you eat, and you could forget about taking a bunch of supplements to survive and thrive? You may be saying, "Man, you're talking crazy stuff, dude. Humans aren't stupid animals. Plus, everyone knows you have to take supplements. I mean, there was, like, evolution and stuff, so we stopped having to behave like animals!"

One day in the future, when we're all walking around in our sexy *Star Trek*–style blue or red unitards and chatting on our tricorders and ordering our food from the teleporter, we'll probably have access to a delicious and completely nutritious superfood that's guaranteed to satisfy us and keep us healthy, happy, and thriving. Currently, I'm doing my best to stay lean so that one day, when sporting that tight little space uniform, I won't have a belly hanging over my belt. (I don't want Captain Kirk to think he needs to send me on one of the away teams as an extra because I'm out of shape. Those guys always get killed!) For now, though, that twenty-third-century magic superfood hasn't been developed. Yet I find that I'm getting similar results by eating something that's not quite so modern.

Could a diet that's just a bunch of meat be healthy? Is it totally crazy? If you tried it, would you die or instantly get sick? Would a lack of fiber lead to an immediate colon mutiny? Stick around and see.

Former interim *New England Journal of Medicine* editor-in-chief Marcia Angell, MD, has been quoted as saying, "It is simply not possible to believe much of the clinical research that has been published or to rely on the judgment of trusted physicians or authoritative medical guidelines. I take no pleasure in this conclusion, which I reached slowly and reluctantly over my two decades as an editor of the *New England Journal of Medicine*." In "Drug Companies & Doctors: A Story of Corruption," Angell explains that our evidence is pretty much bought and paid for. This includes drug companies and the pharmaceuticals they produce as well as nutrition. Unfortunately, disease is big business, and there's not much money in healthy people.

Dr. George Lundberg, a former editor of the *Journal of the American Medical Association*, also has publicly stated that we have screwed up with our nutritional advice and the research around it. He believes that the demonization of fat was never warranted and that the data never really supported the idea that dietary fat is the bad guy. Every single day, more and more people are looking around as they and their loved ones continue to get sicker, fatter, and unhappier, and they realize they've been sold a bill of goods that isn't worth much. We need to reexamine how we look at things.

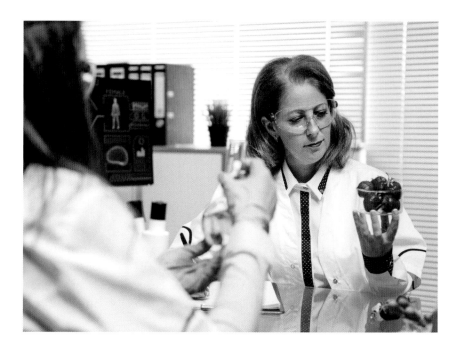

Old Assumptions and New Hypotheses

Okay—if most of our nutritional research is not very helpful, and we've collectively wasted decades of time and incalculable amounts of money, what do we do now? Answer: We start over. *Start over?* Yep, we throw out untested old assumptions, and we start again. What do I mean by old assumptions? Well, let's see.

Assumption	Alternative Hypothesis
All humans thrive on whatever diet they have been observed eating historically.	To survive, humans will eat whatever is available, whether optimal or not.
All humans need certain minimal amounts of vitamins, minerals, and other cofactors regardless of diet.	The requirement for vitamins, minerals, and cofactors vary based upon a person's dietary strategy.
Humans function best on a widely varied diet that includes as many different sources of nutrition as possible.	Humans function best on a high-quality diet of limited variety.
Plants, particularly fruits and vegetables, are a tremendous source of phytonutrients, antioxidants, and essential fiber; thus, we need to eat plenty of them.	There are zero requirements for phytonutrients, antioxidants, and fiber in our diets. They are optional.

You see where I'm going here: We've made lots of assumptions about nutrition, but we haven't formally tested those assumptions. We assume the advice is true and therefore unassailable. When we start over, we need to test these assumptions. Why didn't we do that in the first place?

Eat Your Damn Vegetables!

When we look back at the creation of the modern "science" of nutrition, we can see that the various philosophies are influenced by their founders' beliefs. For example, Lenna Cooper founded the American Dietetic Association (now called the Academy of Nutrition and Dietetics) in 1917. Cooper was a member of the Seventh-day Adventist Church, which encourages a vegetarian lifestyle. Not surprisingly, vegan and vegetarian advocates often quote studies conducted at Loma Linda University, which is supported by the Seventh-day Adventist Church.

When I ask someone what the "truth" is about a topic, the person often looks at me as if I'm some kind of weirdo. I may, in fact, be weird, but that's beside the point, which is that often we don't *know* what the truth is because we consider the "truth" to be whatever we've heard the most. We see this in religion, politics, and nutrition.

Your parents, their parents, and a few generations of great-grandparents probably heard the same refrain as children: "It doesn't matter if you don't like them; eat your veggies because they're good for you." This mantra is in our collective consciousness and has never been challenged; therefore, it must be the truth! The interesting thing is that if you go back only a few hundred years, you'd find that our ancestors thought many vegetables caused illness; guests would have been insulted to have been served veggies at a meal. Throughout much of the world, vegetables, and especially fruits, were rarely consumed. I'm not saying that vegetables and fruits were *always* considered undesirable, but people often went without them in significant quantity. Of course, when I explain this to people, they often reply with, "Oh, yeah? Well, our ancestors didn't live very long, either."

The topic of longevity is probably one of the most misleading subjects in nutrition. We often hear about "Blue Zones" and how people in these areas eat a certain way that enables them to live a long time. We also learn that our prehistoric predecessors lived brutish lives and died incredibly young. Let's tackle the Blue Zone thing first.

Throughout the world, pockets of people have lived a long time eating varied diets that are plant-centric, meat-centric, and well-balanced. We call these areas of longer-than-average life span *Blue Zones*. Unfortunately, diet is only one of the numerous factors that determine life expectancy, and it's not among the top factors. In fact, although a few plant-diet-heavy Blue Zones have been identified, there are numerous populations that we can point to that eat lots and lots of meat *and* live to be very old. For example, residents of Hong Kong consume more meat than just about any other place in the world. Guess what? They live longer than anyone else! (See Figure 2.1.) Does this mean that eating meat makes residents of Hong Kong live a long time? No, we can't say that any more than we can say that eating plants makes Okinawans live a long time. Other factors that influence life span and have a greater impact on longevity than diet include population wealth, water quality, smoking rates, access to care, sanitation, and cultural practices. These factors are among the reasons that the modern Inuit—who live in poverty, smoke at extremely high rates, and have very limited access to healthcare and sanitation—have life spans about ten years shorter than their wealthier neighbors from the same regions. Incidentally, the Inuits' life expectancy in the nineteenth century was pretty much equal to that of the rest of the world, according to census data from the mid-nineteenth century.

Factors That Affect Longevity

GENDER

GENETICS

PRENATAL AND
CHILDHOOD CONDITIONS

MARITAL STATUS

SOCIO-ECONOMIC STATUS

EDUCATION

ETHNICITY/MIGRANT
STATUS

LIFESTYLE

MEDICAL TECHNOLOGY

Even though it's silly to play the longevity game based on diet, sometimes it's fun to do, and believe me, there are people whose entire livelihood depends on it. Let's look at life expectancies of different places in the world and compare them to beef consumption in those areas.

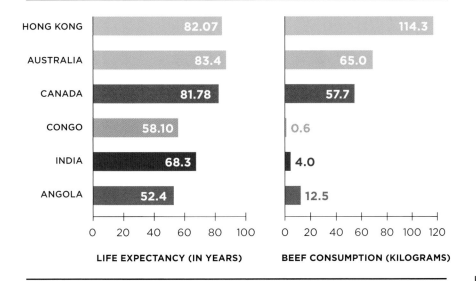

Figure 2.1
Life expectancy in years
(UN data 2010–2015)
and 2016 per capita beef
consumption in
kilograms (FAS/USDA)

Based on this data, we could say that people who eat at least 50 kilograms of beef per year live about fifteen to thirty years longer than those who eat less than 15 kilograms. Of course, anyone with the slightest bit of curiosity would say, "Wait a minute. You compared poor countries to rich countries." Of course, but then I could say that I magically determined that wealth represents a factor of 0.33, and I've made an arbitrary adjustment. Now the "Beef Advantage" is just ten to twenty years. This is how it goes in Cherry Picking Lane, where researchers use the bits of data they need to support their arguments. We see that exact thing happening over and over again with all kinds of nutritional and medical associational studies. The researchers have biases, they measure or select the data they want, and then they make necessary adjustments as they deem fit. I used a rudimentary example; often, more sophisticated methods are employed. Depending upon the beliefs the study is based on, the outcomes can almost always show what you already believe to be true. More often than not, research is done to "prove" an existing assumption or hypothesis rather than to actually test it.

Many hard-working, honest researchers try to conduct their studies without bias, but some researchers have published plenty of studies while having conflicting financial or belief biases. The problem is that we don't know how to determine which studies were bias-free and which weren't. Only recently have researchers been asked to declare biases. Even then the declaration is voluntary, so often researchers don't declare belief-based biases (such as, "I'm a vegan" or "I'm a carnivore").

For the record, I'm decidedly pro-meat and would likely sell my soul for a lifetime supply of steaks! Speaking of which, I'm getting hungry. Time for a rib-eye break. In the next chapter, I talk about some cool anthropology stuff.

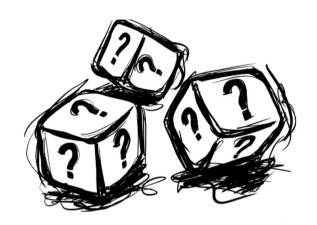

CHAPTER THREE

EVOLUTIONARY GUESSING GAME

As I'm happily sitting here with a belly full of fatty, delicious rib-eye steak and reflecting upon just how primitively satisfying my meal was, I can't help but wonder why that's so. If we go back far enough into our history, I think we'll find clues to this mystery.

If you don't believe that humans evolved or that evolutionary science is real, then just flip ahead and skip this chapter. If, like me, you're fascinated by information about how humans evolved, dig in, and let's try and make some sense of why meat is so satisfying to us.

Hunter Comes Before Gatherer

Let's imagine a prototypical caveman named Urk. He's the strong silent type, but don't mistake him for a dullard. He's intelligent and resourceful, and he wields some incredibly simple but effective technology.

We don't have time-travel technology, and we have only a relatively small number of fossil records, so anything we try to conclude about Urk and our other ancestors from the limited data we have is, at best, highly speculative. As when we rely heavily on nutritional epidemiology, this kind of speculation has the potential for problems. But the bottom line is that almost everything is speculation in the end, so onward with the speculation!

In his excellent book *The Primal Blueprint,* author Mark Sisson used what I think is the best name for a prototypical caveman—Grok—so I had to go with my number-two choice, Urk. *The Primal Blueprint* is a great book about using lifestyle to promote health.

Because we can only speculate about many of the details of our ancestors' habits, we often look to modern hunter-gatherer tribes to make some comparisons. That sometimes leads us to assume that we need to mimic their diets and life-styles because these people tend to be generally free of many of the diseases we associate with the Western lifestyle and diet. Although it's often true that these people aren't obese or sick, they occupy an environmental situation that is almost definitely not what the majority of our ancient ancestors experienced, which means our assumptions may be flawed.

You might be wondering why I don't just skip this speculation and jump right to telling you that you should just eat a damn steak and be done with it. Well, first, anthropology is fun stuff. Second, this information gives you something to talk about as you defend the fact that you like eating steaks.

Most of the indigenous tribes that still inhabit the earth are isolated, primarily in tropical locations. Some indigenous people still live in the cold Arctic regions, but we often dismiss these folks as not relevant because their eating habits tend not to line up with the usual mantra of eating five servings of fruits and vegetables per day. However, if we look at the eras through which the human species evolved, we can see that the average temperature of the earth has been increasing, which means that our ancestors lived in environments that were cooler and drier than what we experience today. In fact, the earth that we inhabit today is far warmer and wetter than at almost any other time our species has roamed the planet. (See Figure 3.1.)

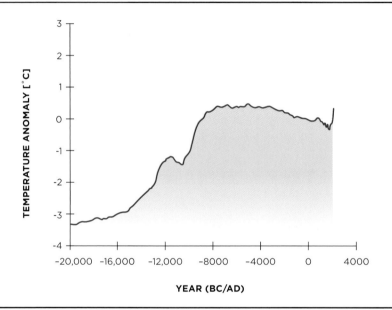

Figure 3.1
Earth's temperature
trend

This cooler, drier situation of the past promoted growth of grasslands more than tropical forests. Humans would have occupied much of these grasslands, and you know what else lived there? Steaks! Big, massive megafaunal animals such as mastodons, elephants, mammoths, aurochs, and woolly rhinoceros were widely distributed throughout Eurasia and Africa. The evidence that we hunted and ate these animals is fairly robust. Archaeologists have found myriad hunting tools throughout the world, and the earliest known art depicts the hunt for large animals. It's very likely that these animals were humans' primary food source and that our ances- tors became highly efficient at finding, killing, and butchering them for the incredibly concentrated and massive amount of nutrition the meat provid- ed. Surprisingly, these giant beasts, whose full-grown size protected them from most predator attacks, were easy pickings for early humans and their basic weapon technology.

Before *Homo habilis* fashioned the first crude stone tools about 2.8 million years ago and became arguably the first "human," earlier hominins had been prowling the African savannas and getting their first taste of meat. Scientists postulate that early prehumans and many archaic humans spent at least a portion of their time as scavengers. In fact, one of the remarkable and unique things about our human digestive tract compared to other primates is our incredibly acidic gastric pH. The stomach acid in a normal, healthy human is around 1.1 to 1.5, which is incredibly acidic and on par with scavenging animals such as the vulture and the hyena. Compare that pH to that of herbivorous primates, which register around 4.0, or even other carnivorous predators, which have a gastric pH of 2 to 3. Maintaining this super acid capacity requires a significant amount of energy resources, and it's not likely that it occurred randomly in humans; there must be a reason for it. That reason is almost certainly that our ancestors needed to deal with pathogens that likely would have been on the food sources (that they scavenged). Interestingly, rabbits, which are herbivores, also have a similarly acidic stomach, possibly because they engage in coprophagy (they eat their own poop!).

Other evidence that humans were once scavengers comes from studies on African lions, which have revealed that the lions often leave a significant amount of meat on a carcass after they've eaten their fill. Often the quantity is enough to feed several hungry humans. Researchers have recorded footage of indigenous African hunters who steal or scavenge meat from a lion's kill. In addition to scavenging, it's very likely that early humans also ate meat that they preserved via various methods—such as drying it in the sun, storing it underwater, or placing it in the snow—that still would have had a significant bacterial load.

One of the oft-discussed topics in nutrition circles is that our ancestors frequently were faced with periods of food scarcity. Therefore, we modern humans should periodically fast for prolonged periods to mimic that situation. Certainly periods of food scarcity existed in our history, and I agree that a constant influx of food every few hours is suboptimal for health for many people. However, it's not clear that early humans, who were surrounded with abundant megafaunal animals and had the technology to kill them easily and then preserve the meat, were going without food often. That situation may have changed when all the big critters went away, and our ancestors had to chase relatively fast, skinny animals to have meat. At that point, they might have had to be more reliant on plants as a food source, which eventually resulted in the development of an agricultural system. With animals being harder to catch and plants subject to the seasonality of growing seasons, our ancestors probably faced more periods of food scarcity. (See Figure 3.2.)

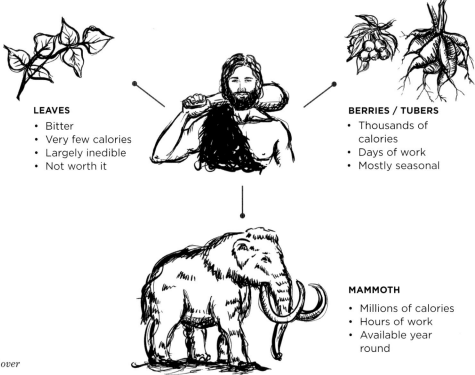

LEAVES
- Bitter
- Very few calories
- Largely inedible
- Not worth it

BERRIES / TUBERS
- Thousands of calories
- Days of work
- Mostly seasonal

MAMMOTH
- Millions of calories
- Hours of work
- Available year round

Figure 3.2
Hunting favored over
gathering

You might be saying, "Surely humans would have eaten various berries, nuts, tubers, and whatnot along the way." Of course, but that doesn't contradict the point of a carnivore diet. Man is an opportunist omnivore and probably a facultative carnivore as well, and the capacity to extract some nutrition from plants was likely a conserved feature from the very first primates.

Let's compare humans with other primates so we can see there's been a dramatic shift in the makeup of the gastrointestinal system. A chimpanzee, for example, has a dramatically larger proportion of its digestive tract dedicated to the cecum and colon and a proportionally smaller percentage of the small intestine. The large intestine and particularly the cecum are specialized to provide fermentation of fibrous plant material to obtain fatty acids via the action of microbes, and an herbivore needs that kind of specialized equipment. The capacity for humans to handle that level of fermentation is dramatically lower than that of chimps and other primates. In humans, the small intestine is where the action occurs for digestion and absorption of meat after the powerful stomach acid does its job further upstream. (See Figure 3.3.)

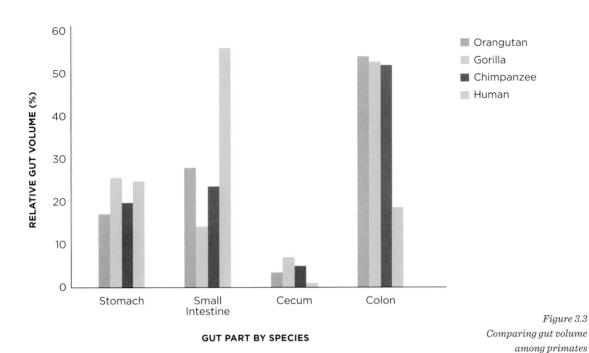

Figure 3.3
Comparing gut volume
among primates

Given the structure of our digestive systems, humans do have some small capacity to extract a minimal amount of calories from fibrous plants. However, relying on only plants to supply our nutritional needs would be a pretty poor strategy, particularly because our brains are such energy hogs. A chimp spends ten more times chewing vegetation than a human does chewing meat to extract the calories and other nutrients from its food, and a gorilla spends even more time chewing. If we look at predictions about early humans based on jaw structure, we can estimate that they spent only about 4 percent of their time chewing, so we can feel pretty safe saying that they weren't munching on leaves and stems all day.

If we look at the gastrointestinal tract anatomy and compare the fermentative capacity of humans to other animals, we find that we're most similar to cats and dogs. These dramatic anatomic adaptations likely occurred in response to millions of years of dietary exposure to copious amounts of meat and relatively small amounts of plant fiber.

Species	Percentage of Digestive Tract Dedicated to Fermentation of Plant Material
Sheep	83
Guinea pit	80
Cattle	75
Horse	69
Gorilla	65
Chimpanzee	60
Rabbit	51
Pig	48
Human	17
Cat	16
Dog	14

Table 3.1
Comparing human and animal digestive tracts

Another popular misconception is that vegetables always have been part of the human diet. (Let me clarify that when I say *vegetable*, I'm referring to the leaves and the stem portions of plants. Fruits, nuts, and root vegetables are a different topic.) You might imagine that prehistoric man was constantly gathering wild broccoli, spinach, or kale to accompany his berries, nuts, and rarely procured piece of meat.

If you go outside and randomly start eating leaves and stems, you'll probably get strange looks from your neighbors. More importantly, you likely will get very sick. Plants get pissed off when we destroy those particular parts of their anatomy; therefore, they protect those areas with toxic and bitter-tasting chemicals. Indeed, the vast majority of plants are toxic for humans to eat. Only through thousands of years of cultivation have we been able to eat any significant amount of vegetables. The other portions of the plants (the fruits, seeds, and roots) also aren't completely benign. I talk more about this stuff later, but for now, I'm just pointing out that stems and leaves were a horrible, bitter-tasting option that would have yielded almost no usable energy for our prehistoric ancestors, and it's very doubtful that early humans would have bothered to eat these plants except in times of utter desperation. Can you imagine the poor dude who was selected to be the plant taster in that situation?

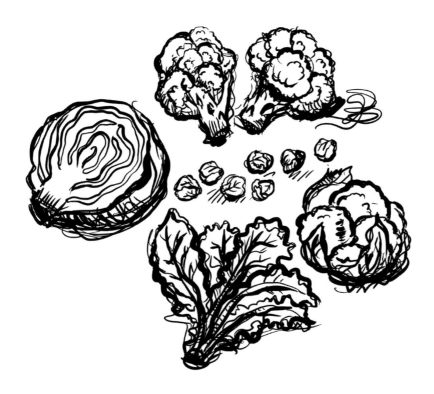

Phytochemicals, cellulose, fiber, micronutrients, chlorophyll, macros—our ancestors didn't know what any of that stuff was, and they couldn't have cared less. They certainly weren't sitting around talking about a balanced diet. What were they looking for? That's simple: protein and calories. Hands down, the most efficient way to meet those needs was to take down a big, fatty, energy-filled megafaunal animal. The amount of time and effort required to obtain the same amount of calories and protein from gathering nuts, fruits, and tubers was greater by at least an order of magnitude. Furthermore, many geographic areas wouldn't have had a reliable year-round source of nonanimal nutrition.

The reason we conquered the planet was the ubiquity of animals. Humans are the greatest predators ever to walk the earth! We aren't successful predators because of pointy teeth, sharp claws, or extreme strength but because of our brains, which are the best weapons on the planet. Our mastery of the environment and our use of effective tools gave us a big leg up on the competition and enabled us to fight above our weight class. Think about it: For every animal that exists, we have figured out a way to eat it. Humans eat birds, bugs, fish, cats, dogs, sharks, whales, llamas, monkeys. You name it; we've eaten it for sure. Even present-day indigenous humans who live in very tropical climates where fruit and other edible plants continuously exist still prioritize hunting animals because they know meat is vital for survival.

Among anthropologists, there's no question that humans have always eaten meat; the only question is how much did we eat. Researchers have found evidence of butchery as far back as a few million years; investigators have found tools that were clearly designed for butchery and hunting, and animal fossils show evidence of cut marks associated with human activity. We've seen countless cave paintings and other artifacts throughout the world that depict large game animals and hunting scenes; they're in all the places we have evidence that man lived. Stable radio isotope data show that in certain areas man was as carnivorous, or perhaps even more carnivorous, than other predators such as wolves.

The brain size of *Homo sapiens* peaked around 100,000 years ago at about 1,500 cubic centimeters (cm³), up from the 400 cm³ of the *Australopithecus*. The vast majority of that brain growth occurred as *Homo sapiens* learned to exploit meat for nutrition but far before we learned to cook. Also, remember that fruit-eating primates have been around for tens of millions of years, and even though they eat the most carbohydrate-energy-rich food available, they haven't made any significant gains in brain size.

As the abundant megafaunal food supply dwindled, out of necessity, our ancestors had to become more reliant on alternative sources of fuel. Some researchers think that a gradual reduction in the elephant population is one of the critical pressures that drove many of the evolutionary adaptations of humans. Instead of hunting big megafauna that we could readily dispatch with a thrusting spear, humans had to get fat from smaller, faster, more agile, and harder-to-track sources. Hunting smaller animals required more complex organizational cooperative efforts, which likely drove developments in speech and intellect. Humans became slenderer, and their skeletons adapted to support long-distance running and hurling projectiles at high velocities. It's likely that our ancestors went to greater efforts to extract as much energy as possible from the fat from the animal kills, such as by extracting bone marrow and using all the fat in and around the organs.

Experts debate the reason that megafaunal animals died off. Most believe it was largely due to overhunting and other human-driven environmental pressures, as evidenced by the fact that in most places megafaunal species became extinct shortly after *Homo sapiens* came on the scene. Alternatively, some experts claim that climate change was a major contributor. Regardless of the reason, megafaunal animals died off, and humans have been under increased pressure to find alternative fuel sources ever since that time.

It's estimated that around 25,000 years ago, the *Homo sapiens* experienced a reduction in robustness, with significant losses in skeletal height, bone thickness, and even 200 cm³ of brain size. Indeed, once we fully adopted agriculture about 10,000 to 12,000 years ago, it becomes very easy to see the difference between the skeleton of a so-called hunter-gatherer and the skeleton of a farmer. The former is much more robust.

What would cause this relative skeletal stunting and overall reduction in brain size? The most likely explanation is a dramatic reduction in overall population nutrition. We often use the average height of a population as a proxy measure for nutritional adequacy. Interestingly, arguably the tallest humans to have ever existed were the Gravettians, a group that lived in central Europe about 30,000 years ago. They were known to be prodigious hunters of mammoths. The estimated average height of males in this group was around 6'2", which is taller than the tallest population in the world today, which is about 6'0".

Farming, particularly growing grains, ultimately allowed for a relatively easily accessible and cheap source of calories to fuel an ever-expanding population. Our ancestors didn't conduct randomized controlled trials before collectively deciding to increase their dependence on grains; they largely did not have a choice, and that's been the case ever since. When there's no more mammoth meat and lots of mouths to feed, you need to make more grain, learn to cultivate more fruit, and eventually even convert some of those toxic and bitter-tasting leaves and stems into something edible called vegetables. They got better and more efficient at extracting energy from tubers, nuts, and seeds, so they cultivated them to produce greater yields of energy, less fibrous material, and fewer toxins, and they also figured out how to eliminate or decrease the toxic chemicals in those foods through ingenious methods of preparation—soaking, sprouting, fermenting, and cooking. The foods that people likely had used sparingly (or not at all) during the days of abundant megafauna became frequent menu options.

Today the situation is even worse. Now we have toxic vegetable oils, which were introduced to the human diet about 120 years ago, high-fructose corn syrup, artificial flavors, cereals with brightly colored marshmallows, and so forth. We've tried to replace fundamental human nutrition with a constant stream of new flavors, shapes, color combinations, supplements, and additives. We've turned a basic human function into a form of entertainment and addiction, and we're certainly no better for it. Remember, humans are opportunists. If junk foods had been available 50,000 years ago, our ancestors definitely would have eaten that garbage, too.

Surely, though, we're better than those lowly cavepeople were, right? We've all heard the claims that prehistoric man lived a short, painful existence capped off at about age thirty. As an orthopedic surgeon, I've often wondered how the heck someone can tell how old people were from looking at skeletons from 50,000 years ago. It's fairly easy to identify the approximate age of a kid; if you show me the X-ray of a child, I can generally tell you what age they are plus or minus a year. It's harder to

If junk foods had been available 50,000 years ago, our ancestors definitely would have eaten that garbage, too.

estimate for adults. In fact, many anthropologists agree that after a person reaches a certain age, there isn't a good way to identify the age based only on the skeleton, so they often say thirty to forty years without knowing exactly how long someone lived. So, it's possible that those early humans made it to seventy or even eighty. We assume dental, bone, and joint wear patterns then were the same as they are now, and that assumption certainly may not be valid. Infant mortality data also is a factor in the life expectancy data, and that can skew the average life expectancy. For example, say you have two skeletons. One is two years old, and one is eighty years old. We would say that the overall life expectancy of that group was only forty-one years [(2 + 80 years) / 2 people = 41 years].

So, Urk was running around with his relatively big brain, getting plenty of food by eating big, fatty-meat-filled animals, migrating across the world, perhaps eating a berry here and there, and likely thriving. From a nutritional standpoint, that same situation has never again existed in human history until today. Now, the 25,000 years of relative animal drought has finally been reversed via modern agricultural efficiency and population wealth. And although we can no longer obtain fatty mammoth meat, the closest proxy we have on a commercial scale is the cow, and we have become very efficient at producing them. Yes, it's harsh to talk about animals as food, but ultimately that is what they are

We live in a world of relative ease and comfort. We can tap a few buttons on our phones to make food suddenly appear, as if by magic. We take for granted that we can get food from all over the world at any time of the year. We are used to 100 flavors of ice cream, 25 kinds of potato chips, strawberries the size of our fists, and bananas in January in Canada. That's today's reality, but it's who we've adapted to be—not who we've always been. The grim reality is that we aggressively ate other animals. We devoured their flesh daily; we understood who we were, and, honestly, it's who we still are.

Historical Clues

What can observations about historical populations tell us? I think that we can use them to talk about possibilities, but it's a mistake to think that our ancestors did everything perfectly. Yes, when trying to provide evidence in support of a carnivore diet, we can point to successful multigenerational populations like the Maasai, Inuit, and Mongolians. Some interesting data comes from accounts of those cultures, and many people who are vocal proponents of a carnivore diet point to these ancient peoples as proof of concept and will often attempt to emulate them.

Can humans survive on just meat? I think the answer is clearly yes. Are there some special genetic adaptations or a unique situation that allowed only certain populations to do it? I think that question plays into a bias that we have been taught to believe about nutrition. We see it all the time. "The only way the Inuit were able to avoid scurvy was because they all ate some berries or muktuk, or they ate raw meat or lots of organs. Therefore, we must do that as well." Many of those assumptions did not even apply to all Inuit, and it's also extremely easy to point out plenty of people today that don't do any of those things and yet are thriving (yours truly, for example).

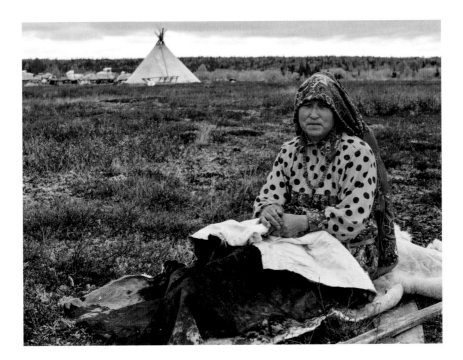

Although we don't need to replicate exactly what these cultures have been doing to thrive, we can learn some interesting things from them. For example, the Maasai, who spend a significant portion of their lives eating nothing but meat and drinking blood and milk, don't show any signs of scurvy or any other vitamin or mineral deficiency. They haven't been constantly plagued with gastrointestinal problems as a result of some plant fiber deficiency. They haven't gone blind or crazy or suffered in any way due to a lack of plant phytonutrients or exogenous plant antioxidants. The same could be said of other cultures in the northern hemisphere, who do not share the exact genetics of the Maasai.

In fact, all over the world, there have been accounts of populations that have thrived on fully carnivore diets (or on diets that are almost entirely meat based). Despite our differences, we are all the same species, and we all can eat the same food and thrive provided that food is meat.

As humans started to introduce more variety into their diets, we've begun to see some minor differences in tolerance of other foods. A classic example is lactose intolerance. People often ask me about the "blood type" diet, in which you're supposed to eat certain foods based on your blood type. I always say that if your blood is red, you have the right blood type to eat meat. It's that simple, even though that idea runs counter to the current trend of personalized medicine based on each person's genetic makeup. Everyone is a special snowflake, but we are all the same species.

Let's talk about some of the disparate groups of people who've largely subsisted on meat and thrived. The Yeoman Warders of England, who are also known as the Beefeaters, were hand-picked guardians of the royalty. It's believed that they were called *Beefeaters* because they received large rations of beef, possibly as a way to enhance their strength and stamina. During their expedition to explore the American frontier, Lewis and Clark and their companions consumed prodigious amounts of meat—up to nine pounds daily—to fuel their activities. Traditional rural Mongolians have been routinely noted to consume ten pounds of meat in one sitting, and a few together could consume an entire sheep in a single day. The largest empire to ever exist was that of Genghis Kahn. His army, which conquered vast swathes of Asia and Europe, relied on a diet that was almost completely meat-based.

Similarly, the Gauchos of Southern Brazil and Argentina were known to spend long periods consuming meat-only diets. At one point in ancient Greece, there was a bit of a carnivore movement, and some of the original Olympic athletes were using meat-based diets to excel. The Nenets of northern Russia and the Sámi of northern Scandinavia have traditionally survived almost exclusively on reindeer, although the Sámi also added fish and some occasional berries to their diet.

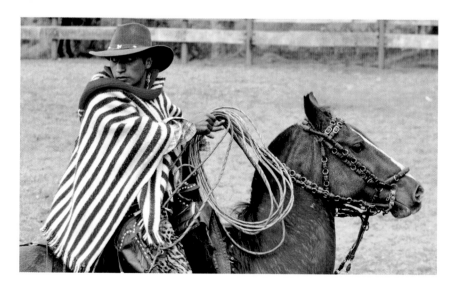

Meat-Based Diet Pioneers

I didn't invent this diet. Aside from historical populations, some individuals have preceded me in suggesting that a meat-based diet is the way to go. Credit for being the "inventor" of the diet probably goes to some *Australopithecus* dude who lived four million years ago—possibly Urk's great-grandfather 1,000 times removed. More recently, though, some physicians and scientists have advocated for a carnivore diet.

- Dr. James Salisbury, whose legacy lives on via Salisbury steak (of TV dinner fame), believed that the human digestive tract was most suited for meat and that humans did best by avoiding fruits, vegetables, and starches to prevent toxins from causing various ailments such as heart disease, tumors, and mental health problems.

- Arctic explorer Vilhjalmur Stefansson's *The Fat of the Land* is often cited as a reference in favor of all-meat diets.

- Dr. Blake Donaldson published *Strong Medicine* in 1962. In it, he described how he used a meat-based diet in his practice for decades with remarkable success.

- Gastroenterologist Walter Voegtlin wrote the 1972 book *The Stone Age Diet* in which he proclaims that any human who wasn't able to adapt to survive upon a diet of just fatty meat rapidly died off.

- Dr. H. L. Newbold also focused on a carnivore approach in his 1991 book *Type A/Type B Weight Loss Book*.

- Even Dr. Robert Atkins promoted an approach that was largely meat-based, particularly during the "induction phase" of his eponymous diet.

So, by no means is this carnivore diet a new thing. Certainly, the diet will be labeled as faddish, and many people will try it out before deciding it's not for them. But there's a reason this approach keeps coming around. Each time it resurfaces, we're dealing with a progressively sicker population than the last time the diet received attention.

One thing is significantly different today than during the other eras when my predecessors promoted a meat-based diet: We now have interconnectedness like no other time in human history. Today, via the power of the Internet, we no longer have to rely on the powers that be to tell us what research suggests we should do. Today we can instantly access hundreds, if not thousands, of people who are in situations similar to our own, and we can start to conclude what may be effective for us. People who are used to the traditional method of receiving information that's meted out in a rigorously controlled fashion are very disturbed by this new paradigm.

We can see real results in real people to whom we can talk to get answers to our questions. The power to amass knowledge and data is amplified exponentially compared to traditional means. When something works well, it starts to spread throughout the community. Early adopters test the system. They find holes and figure out patches for them. This system is possibly a far more effective system than anything else, and I think its potential is just now being tapped. Of course, we'll see a great deal of pushback and a lot of attempts at fear mongering and vilification from mainstream nutrition advocates. Fortunately, an educated populace is starting to be able to see past that kind of naysaying.

Now take another Steak Break. In the next chapter, I get into some of the common myths about why a diet like this is supposedly dangerous.

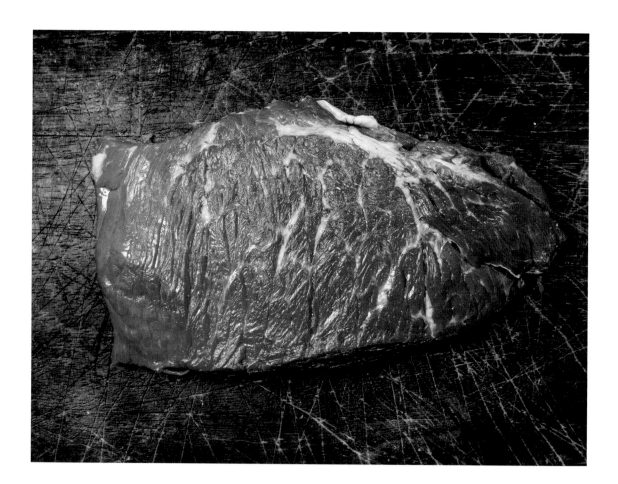

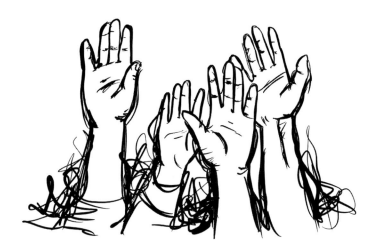

CHAPTER FOUR

ADDRESSING
THE QUESTIONS

When I first embarked on my crazy journey into carnivory, I heard from all sorts of naysayers and prophets of doom. They'd always say, "But what about scurvy or other deficiencies?" or, "But what about clogged arteries? Or what if you don't poop without fiber? Or what if your microbiome revolts?" On and on it went.

Just as with the numerous historical populations who've lived this kind of lifestyle for decades (or longer), none of those things have happened to me. My teeth haven't fallen out because of scurvy, my heart hasn't clogged up, and I've been going to the bathroom just fine. In fact, my digestion has been the best it's ever been. How can all this be true? I wondered the same thing. It was almost as if a lot of the modern nutritional teachings were wrong!

In this chapter, I go over some of the common misconceptions and fallacies about eating an all-meat diet and explain why some of the common beliefs don't hold up in actual practice.

What About Vitamin and Mineral Deficiencies?

Let's look at some science to help us to feel good by examining what we can observe. Do people on carnivore diets develop scurvy, which is a deadly result of vitamin C deficiency? Basically, the answer is a resounding no. The one exception would be if you attempted to live off a diet of only dried and preserved meats. That type of diet is the reason British sailors developed scurvy. For months at a time, they lived off dried, salted meats while they traveled the sea. High-carbohydrate items comprised the rest of their diets, and those foods potentially made matters worse.

Let's take a minute to discuss what vitamin C does. It has numerous roles in the body. One role is to assist in the synthesis of collagen, which is a vital protein used structurally throughout the body. When collagen synthesis is down, we see some of the classic symptoms of scurvy, such as bleeding gums, loss of teeth, joint dysfunction, and nonhealing wounds. The body also uses vitamin C to help form carnitine, and vitamin C acts as an antioxidant that plays a role in modulating our immune systems. Humans who are deficient in vitamin C start to show signs of scurvy within a few months. However, I've been eating only meat for a couple of years, and I've only gotten stronger. Unless increased strength is a rare, previously unrecognized symptom of scurvy, I'm not suffering from a lack of vitamin C.

Okay, so if vitamin C is necessary, meat doesn't contain vitamin C (at least according to the U.S. Department of Agriculture), and humans can't make vitamin C, what gives? Why are so many people who follow an all-meat diet not walking around with their teeth falling out? Well, several things are in play.

It has been known for well more than 100 years that meat, particularly fresh meat, both cures and prevents scurvy. This evidence was well documented among many nineteenth-century Arctic explorers. Fresh meat is the key difference in a modern carnivore's diet compared to the diets of the British sailors, which was dominated by dried, salted meat. Amber O'Hearn, a brilliant long-term carnivore, investigated the USDA's claim that meat has no vitamin C. She was shocked to discover that the USDA had never bothered to test for vitamin C in meat. As it turns out, meat does contain a small but sufficient amount of the vitamin, particularly in the context of a fully carnivore diet.

Vitamin C enters your body through the intestinal tract. Interestingly, glucose can directly compete with vitamin C absorption because they share a cellular transporter. If there's a lot of glucose in your system, vitamin C absorption is effectively inhibited. In a meat-only diet, glucose is effectively zero in the intestines; thus, vitamin C becomes more available. Interesting work coming out of the Paleo Medicina group in Hungary has shown that serum vitamin C levels are normal in patients who follow a carnivore diet. In fact, animal-derived vitamin C was more effective than similar plant-derived vitamin C for maintaining serum levels.

Dietary antioxidants are widely believed to benefit us, although there are some significant challenges to that theory that I discuss later in this book. As I mentioned previously, vitamin C has a role here. It's interesting to note that when an animal that can manufacture its own vitamin C starts eating a carbohydrate-restricted diet, the animal's synthesis of vitamin C decreases. It's almost as if eating carbohydrates *increases* the requirements for antioxidants. Although humans can't make vitamin C as other animals can, in the presence of a low-carbohydrate diet, we see an increase in some of our endogenous antioxidants (that is, our body makes them).

The role of vitamin C in helping to form collagen involves the hydroxylation of the amino acids proline and lysine to form hydroxyproline and hydroxylysine, respectively. When you eat a meat-rich diet, some of those molecules are absorbed in the already hydroxylated form via specific gut transporters; therefore, you likely require less vitamin C.

The upshot is that when you're on an all-meat diet, vitamin C absorption is more efficient, and your body's requirements for it go down. You get a sufficient amount of the vitamin from the food (meat) you eat, and you don't get scurvy.

This brings up an interesting point. When officials at the USDA came up with the recommended daily allowances (RDA), they primarily studied populations and individuals who consumed high-carb, grain-based diets. In a 2007 Institute of Medicine review of the RDA, several speakers asserted that the Dietary Reference Indices should be based on a higher standard of evidence than what had been used to formulate the recommendations. Basically, the RDAs are more or less a guess, and they certainly weren't formulated by evaluating people who were eating low-carb or (heaven forbid!) meat-only diets. Consequently, we have no real idea of what the optimal or even sufficient levels of vitamins and minerals are for various subsets of dieters. For now, the entire dietary profession uses this low-quality evidence for the basis of almost all the current recommendations.

We've seen evidence of other differences in requirements for some vitamins, minerals, and cofactors. A deficiency of thiamine, for example, leads to a condition called *beriberi*, which results in severe neurological and cardiac disease. Researchers have found that an animal's requirements for thiamine vary based on that animal's carbohydrate consumption. This result was observed as far back as the late 1800s when scientists noted that

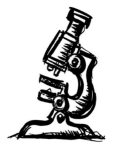

animals fed a low-carbohydrate diet didn't develop disease in the presence of low thiamine levels, but animals fed a high-carbohydrate diet developed disease at the same low thiamine levels.

Magnesium is a mineral that's crucial for many human physiologic functions. Recently magnesium deficiency has been implicated as a potential source of numerous disease states. Interestingly, magnesium is a cofactor that is crucially involved in carbohydrate metabolism, and there is some research showing a relationship between blood glucose and magnesium levels. Is it possible that many people are identified as having a magnesium deficiency because of increased demand via high rates of carbohydrate ingestion? It's certainly an interesting question, and that relationship would account for the lack of any clinically relevant nutrient deficiencies in our observations of the modern-day carnivore-dieter population.

Unfortunately, it's challenging to make assessments about vitamin or mineral deficiencies. We can look for overt clinical symptoms and more subtle subclinical things like poor energy, sleep, or mood. Aside from those symptoms, we're often limited to studying the things we can measure most easily, which generally comes down to a blood test. For all the billions of dollars we spend annually on blood tests, the sad fact is that many are poor predictors of chronic issues. Sure, sometimes we can get important information from a blood test, but to think that a blood serum vitamin C level can tell us something specific, such as the cellular concentration of the vitamin C level in our left tibia, is misguided. Perhaps at steady state, when no environmental or internal changes are occurring, a certain level can be expected to exist, but the truth is that trafficking of materials in the blood can vary wildly. Does sleep, exercise, recent meals, temperature, time of year, injury, or illness (not to mention thousands of other things) affect those concentrations? Almost certainly, the answer is yes. Another solution for identifying problems is to biopsy the tissues, which gives a far better representation of one's nutritional state. The problem is that biopsies often are fairly painful, they require far more risk, and they're expensive. Thus, we continue to rely on unreliable guesswork to make many of our decisions about how to address health issues.

One of the recurring themes that I like to talk about is that, despite what many people like to proclaim, the science of nutrition is *not* settled. (Stating that science is settled would completely undermine the basic concept of science.) Take this theory, for example: Red meat causes diabetes. The evidence in support of this theory would be based on population survey data that shows that people who eat more red meat have higher rates of diabetes. There's nothing wrong with that theory as long as the data continues to support that claim. However, what if you have information to the contrary—such as numerous accounts of people who eat *only* red meat and notice that their diabetes resolves? At this point, you have to adjust

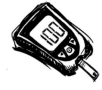

your hypothesis and modify your theory. You could say that maybe it was some other factor common to those meat eaters with diabetes that caused the disease; in other words, maybe meat combined with something else is to blame. Unfortunately, we live in a time when entire industries and careers are built upon a particular hypothesis, and even in the face of new or overwhelming evidence, some people are unwilling to revisit or revise their original assumptions. This is human nature and to be expected. The unfortunate part is that those assumptions can affect many lives around the world, and many billions of dollars are tied up in it.

Here's a general question to ponder before we go on: Why is it that every wild animal that eats meat as part of its diet doesn't suffer from the chronic diseases that modern humans do? How can a food source that is ubiquitous throughout the animal kingdom and has been clearly eaten by humans for millions of years now suddenly be toxic to only humans while every other animal is just fine?

What About Cholesterol?

Let's look at cholesterol, which has enjoyed the status of being the number-one dietary supervillain for at least the past 50 years. Our interpretation of its role has gone through a dramatic change over the last several decades. The fact that we're still unsure what cholesterol's functions are and what significance low and high levels may mean should indicate that we still have a very long way to go to full understanding.

Common wisdom regarding cholesterol, whether total or LDL cholesterol, has been that if it's high, you're at increased risk for cardiovascular disease. Certainly, there is a great deal of scientific theory to back that up. Much of the research comes from associational studies that look at populations and compare rates of heart disease with corresponding cholesterol levels. The evidence includes a number of animal studies, and drug trials have demonstrated that lowering cholesterol can decrease the incidence of disease. Many of these studies have been repeated multiple times with similar results; therefore, perhaps the theory should stand. Indeed, often when someone's blood test comes back with an elevated cholesterol level, the doctor almost automatically offers a drug to lower cholesterol. Heck, I remember when I was a medical student many years ago, I often overheard the attending physicians joking about how popular cholesterol-lowering statin drug Lipitor should be placed in the water supply because all the lazy, fat patients needed to be on it. That's how commonplace treating high cholesterol with drugs had become.

So, let me make a simple observation about conclusions that come from an associational study. Let's assume you have a study that says people with elevated levels of cholesterol have a higher risk of heart disease. Fair enough—certainly there's data to support that. But what if you ask, "Does that association hold up in all people in all situations?" That's a simple question, but it drives a lot of thought and gets at the heart of some of the problems with this type of science. Suppose I could gather a subset of people who have elevated cholesterol but who also are profoundly insulin sensitive; they're also very lean and have low levels of systemic and vascular inflammation. Does the association still hold? Or if it does, is it so small, in light of those other factors, that it's rendered insignificant?

Let's use some arbitrary numbers and say that risk of heart disease goes up 20 percent if you have an LDL higher than 130, but it goes down 150 percent if your insulin is lower than 3. Heart disease goes down another 85 percent if your waist is smaller than your height, and it goes down a further 120 percent if you have a C-reactive protein (a marker of inflammation) level lower than 1.0. In this theoretical situation, your risk for heart disease would be very favorable in the big picture. Now, many would be tempted to suggest that we should lower the risk even more by getting the cholesterol down by using drugs or perhaps a low-fat diet. Certainly, that strategy might be beneficial if all the other factors also remain favorable. But what happens if they don't? What happens if going on the low-fat diet causes your insulin to rise or your C-reactive protein to go up? What happens if you take a drug and the side effects cause you to gain weight, and your waist expands? Those are questions we need to ask.

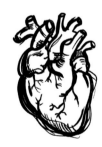

Also, we have a mounting pile of evidence that shows that heart disease risk is more influenced by other factors, including things like hyperinsulinemia, inflammatory status, and triglyceride levels, than it is by cholesterol levels. One interesting group of people that have been studied are those who have a genetic variant that leads to something called *familial hypercholesterolemia*. Basically, many of these people walk around with sky-high cholesterol levels, but they don't die of heart disease any more frequently than anyone else; people with this condition have normal life expectancies. If they have unfavorable insulin levels, the story is different: heart attack city. This implies that high cholesterol by itself is insufficient to cause cardiovascular disease, which should be no surprise because we are complex systems that are affected by myriad interrelated variables.

Dave Feldman, a wonderful citizen scientist, has been demonstrating that our cholesterol levels can change by up to 100 points in a matter of a few days based on nothing more than what that person has eaten in the preceding few days. An interesting study shows that cholesterol rises by about 36 percent when a person fasts for one week. Now, under the assumption that meat is bad for us because it can cause cholesterol to rise (which it can) then does that also mean that eating nothing is equally bad for us?

The assumption is that low cholesterol is always a good thing when it comes to preventing heart disease; because heart disease is our number-one killer, that's where our focus should be. Plus, we have some pretty cool drugs that lower cholesterol and are worth billions of dollars. (But I'm sure no one was concerned about the money to be made from those drugs, right?) However, what about the role of cholesterol outside the discussion of heart disease? What part does it play in our bodies? What effect does it have on things like all-cause mortality? What about diseases like cancer and certain neurodegenerative diseases? Entire books are dedicated to this stuff, but I'll touch on it briefly here. (Believe me, I really want to get back to talking about steaks, but I need to at least mention this stuff.)

Your entire body—every single cell you have—contains cholesterol. That's the major difference between defining a plant cell and an animal cell. (I used to laugh when I'd see advertisements on plant products pointing out the fact that they were "cholesterol free." Well, duh; of course—because they're plants.) Your brain uses something like 25 percent of your body's cholesterol, and many of your hormones are made from it. Cholesterol is integral to the structure of every cell in your body. You can easily find studies that link low cholesterol to depression, violence, suicide, and neurodegenerative diseases. Some studies report that people tend to die younger if they have low cholesterol. Some cancers have been linked to low cholesterol. Infectious disease can be more difficult to fight when cholesterol levels are low.

If you list some of the major associative factors that are believed to be a contributor to heart disease, you will find the relative effect of cholesterol level to be relatively lower on that list. If you then stratified those factors by things that can be most efficiently adjusted with drugs rather than through lifestyle changes, you would see cholesterol at the top of that list. Not surprisingly, billions of dollars have been focused on the factor that's drug-modifiable, whereas the lifestyle factors largely receive lip service.

Suffice it to say that I don't think that low cholesterol is necessarily a good thing. High cholesterol may be problematic in certain cases, but that doesn't necessarily mean it always is. Some people will continue to be concerned about this particular particle or that particular subfraction of this or that lipid, and perhaps that concern and the knowledge it spawns will lead to the answer to immortality. Or perhaps we'll just replace heart disease with cancer, dementia, or some other equally awful way to die. The bottom line is this: You and I will likely die of heart disease or cancer regardless of the diet we choose. For example, data on vegan and vegetarian mortality indicates the number-one and number-two killers for that group are cancer and heart disease. Heart disease kills a lot of people, and most people die with so-called normal cholesterol.

It saddens me to see almost daily that so many people are examined with a simple annual blood lipid test and then offered a drug to lower their cholesterol based only on that test and no further investigation. The overprescribing of cholesterol medications largely comes down to a lack of time and education on the part of physicians. You can literally walk into your doctor's office after having lost every ounce of fat on your body, feeling the best you have in decades, sporting excellent blood pressure and otherwise perfect metabolic markers, but if your annual blood test reveals high cholesterol, you'll still leave the office with a prescription for some medication without any further discussion. In my view, that's unacceptable, and it's a sign of systemic laziness. We have to remember that our physiology is an incredibly complex system with far more going on than we can hope to find out with a snapshot of what's traveling in our blood at one particular instant.

Today, it's encouraging to see more and more patients challenging some of the knee-jerk reaction of their doctors, and the patients are asking for more information. Remember that no one has more at stake regarding your health than you do. Be a pain in the ass; ask for more details and more testing. Challenge your physician to up his game. I've learned more from patients than I ever learned from any textbook.

What About Pooping?

Now let's talk about fiber. The message we've heard for what seems like eons is, "If you don't eat fiber, you can't have a healthy bowel movement." We've been told that fiber is essential for a healthy gut and healthy digestion; the latest word is that it's necessary for a healthy microbiome. There are certainly studies and theories to support these assertions, but I can easily point out many observations that run completely contrary to those theories.

For instance, many carnivorous mammals have no problem whatsoever having normal, regular bowel movements in the complete or nearly complete absence of fiber. For example, my dogs poop on the grass every day despite eating nothing but meat. (I sometimes wish that lack of fiber would prevent them from pooping; then I wouldn't always have to carry those little black dog poop bags every time I go out.) I know what you're saying, and you're right: Humans aren't dogs, and we're not carnivores (maybe), so perhaps we shouldn't compare ourselves to dogs. But we can look to numerous human populations that have had no difficulties with elimination despite living on diets that are essentially devoid of fiber.

For example, I don't recall the early Arctic explorers having to administer enemas to the Inuit populations when they arrived. Perhaps the handful of berries the Inuits would occasionally eat in the summer was sufficient for keeping them regular throughout the rest of the year. Instead of speculating, though, we can ask people today what happens when they go without fiber for a long period. The resounding response is that they have no problem whatsoever having bowel movements. They're regular and comfortable, and most report their overall gastrointestinal function is the best it's ever been in their lives. We have studies showing both that chronic constipation is relieved when the diet contains zero fiber and that people who eat lots of fiber have much higher rates of diverticular disease.

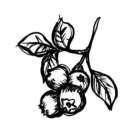

Why do we ignore these observations and instead rely on that good ol' standby of nutritional epidemiology? Could it be because the origins of the nutrition field were tied to vegetarianism and a religious group that started feeding people cereal to cure them from having and acting on impure sexual thoughts? Companies like Kellogg's and other grain-heavy megacompanies continue to influence nutritional organizations via funding of research and support of some of the dietitians' groups. The refrain is, "Eat your fiber, keep your colon nice and full, poop three times a day, and feed those fiber-starved little bacteria." I've heard several prominent vegan proponents state that humans should have an average of three bowel movements per day and should expect to fart fairly frequently because it's a normal state of affairs. They contend that early humans didn't mind passing gas because they spent a lot of time outdoors. As far as I can tell, they pulled this theory out of their vegan asses. You will receive zero prizes at the end of your life for having had the largest bowel movements (in either size or quantity).

You shouldn't be walking around with bloated guts and feeling the need to fart all day long. Why the hell would we have been designed to have a digestive system that caused us pain and discomfort? The short answer is that we weren't. One of the most common "side effects" of a carnivore diet is the near-complete absence of gas. Yes, most people on an all-meat diet stop farting. I know some folks may find this fact a downside because they're quite proud of the fact that they can level a room with relative ease via their methane retro cannon, but I hope most people consider the lack of gas to be an asset of the diet.

As I discussed earlier, fiber reportedly can lower cholesterol; that's great, but I also mentioned that low cholesterol is linked to other conditions, such as dementia, depression, and perhaps cancer. Humans cannot digest fiber because our digestive tract wasn't designed for fiber. Just because we shove fiber-filled foods down our digestive tube and some bacteria start to grow and eat it in no way indicates that our bodies require it. Think of it this way: If we were to start eating dirt, we'd have colons full

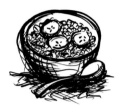

of bacteria that prefer dirt. And if we believed that dirt was good for us, we could most likely find some compound that those dirt-eating bacteria produced that would be of benefit to us. However, if we looked hard enough, we also could find compounds that were detrimental to us. Earlier in the book, I talked about bias in research, and studies about dietary fiber are one place where we can see some bias. Some researchers believe that fiber is good for humans because of some crappy epidemiology. Therefore, they look for beneficial compounds that result from eating fiber while ignoring negative compounds. Can anyone say how a bunch of methane is benefiting our colon? What about the fact that fiber consumption has been shown to increases rates of diverticular disease, or that removing it from the diet often solves longstanding constipation?

Fiber can limit a glucose excursion; for example, if you drink apple juice, you see a fairly typical high spike in postprandial blood glucose, which arguably is a bad thing. If you eat a fiber-rich apple, you get a much lower spike. Well, guess what. If your diet is a bunch of meat, you also avoid large postprandial spikes of glucose. Why would Urk and the rest of our megafauna-munching ancestors have gone out of their way to eat a bunch of fibrous foods that would have provided next to no calories, would have been difficult to digest, and likely would have tasted like cardboard. He didn't have the American Diabetes Association telling him to eat his heart-healthy whole grains and leafy vegetables, which incidentally weren't even cultivated yet. Urk was living it up on the bounty of fatty, delicious meat. From time to time he may have had something a little bit sweet, like some berries, but I can't see him going out of his way to chew on super fibrous roots and bitter leaves unless he was desperate. I know I sure as hell wouldn't have unless I'd had some overzealous dietitian yapping at me about phytonutrients, eating the rainbow, and the ill-defined balanced diet. How the hell do you make a balanced diet when you're living through an ice age?

In the movie *Jerry Maguire*, you might remember that the athlete played by actor Cuba Gooding, Jr. repeatedly yelled, "SHOW ME THE MONEY!" during his contract negotiation. I bring that up here because I don't see any evidence of the doom and gloom reports about poor gut function, scurvy, and micronutrient deficiencies when I look at the real-world application of the carnivore diet. So I have to say, "SHOW ME THE MONEY!" to all the critics. Results are what count. When someone tells me that lack of fiber leads to poor gut health, I say, "How? Show me what the clinical consequences are." All I see is people who report vastly improved digestion and often state that they feel the best they've felt in their lives. People with irritable bowel syndrome or inflammatory bowel disease tend to get better. If that's the case, how does that translate to worsening gut health? I'm just a dumb ol' MD, but that doesn't seem to make sense to me.

My critics would point out that I'm citing anecdotes, the implication being that if anecdotal data doesn't match our preconceived ideas, those reports must be discounted. How about we don't discount this stuff and instead actually listen to our patients rather than our pharmaceutical sponsors?

The more I learn about nutrition, the more I'm convinced that is has its basis in religion as much as it does in science. Think about it: When people become passionate about diet, they often feel strong cultural and ethical emotions. I constantly am amazed at how certain camps get so entrenched about long-held beliefs of what's healthy to eat. It's very different than many other topics. For example, if we were to talk about the science of building furniture, most people wouldn't get too excited because very few people are emotionally invested in whether something is made of cherry or maple. But when we talk about whether we should eat a steak or a big bowl of veggies, people become very animated.

What About Kidney Health and Gout?

People who are emotionally invested in avoiding protein often state that protein damages the kidneys, particularly when that protein comes from animals. Where did this theory come from? Not from studying humans. On the podcast I share with ultra-endurance world-record holder, Zach Bitter, I was talking with Dr. Stuart Phillips, one of the world's leading protein experts, and we got into this topic. The misconception about this issue evolved from some work researchers did on rats, but no research on humans has ever shown the same results.

Protein doesn't damage kidneys, but damaged kidneys tend to leak protein, which is something that contributes to the confusion about the relationship between protein and the kidneys. Many physicians have bought into this myth that protein damages kidneys even though the assertion has almost no scientific support. As with other misconceptions, you can look at the treasure trove of nutritional epidemiology and find some relationship between a high-protein diet and an increased incidence of kidney disease, but, as always, you have to ask the question, "Does it apply to all people in all situations?" In my experience, people who eat a high-protein carnivore diet aren't finding that their kidneys are compromised. I'm not saying that no one who follows the carnivore diet will ever have kidney problems; they can occur for many reasons. But I do not think that an all-meat diet *causes* kidney issues. I know of some cases where chronic kidney dysfunction has started to get better for several people.

Let's put this in perspective. Humans evolved in an environment where eating copious amounts of meat was likely a common occurrence. We have several historical accounts of humans consuming very large amounts of meat, and those accounts show no evidence that the people experienced kidney problems. As I mentioned earlier, the explorers on the Lewis and Clark expedition were noted to have eaten as much as 9 pounds of meat per day. Modern-day competitive eaters have sometimes eaten more than 20 pounds of meat in one sitting without damaging their kidneys. If protein did indeed damage our kidneys, humans would not have made it this far through history.

Another common myth about the consumption of meat is that it leads to the development of gout. This perception goes back to the days when gout was considered a "rich man's" disease. Because the financially well off were diagnosed with gout more frequently than the less affluent population, and the rich also were the people who could afford to eat meat, the assumption was that meat was the cause of gout. However, what do you think we find when we look at people who eat only meat? They don't get gout, and if they had it before they start the carnivore diet, the gout generally clears up.

One of the beautiful things about a carnivore diet is that it tends to make some things crystal clear. You can wallow around in pointless epidemiology or use some questionably applicable animal studies to try to interpret something about the effects of eating meat, or you can take the simpler route and look at people who eat only meat. When we look at populations of meat eaters, such as the Maasai, Mongols, or Sámi, we see that there's no indication that they were hobbled by gout. Today I routinely observe people with gout who go on an all-meat diet; for them, gout becomes a distant memory within months.

So what about those rich dudes from a few hundred years ago? Why did they have gout? Because they had access to something that the common folk did not. Sugar! The wealthy also had more access to alcohol, and both sugar and alcohol are strong drivers of gout. The traditional view of gout is that it's caused by an increase in uric acid because we can see uric acid crystals when we view gouty tissue under a microscope. I've taken care of plenty of gout patients over the years, and I've even removed large gouty tophi (which are basically giant blobs of crystal deposits in the skin that resemble toothpaste when cut open) from all parts of the body. None of my gout-afflicted patients has said he was a pure carnivore. We know that purines form as food breaks down, and they can lead to increased uric acid production. Meat is often high in purines, and thus experts concluded that meat was the reason for the rich man's disease. The problem is that *most* food leads to purines being produced, and high uric acid levels do not always lead to gout. As with all things, the path to gout isn't a simple route. Is uric acid more of a problem when an underlying inflammatory state exists?

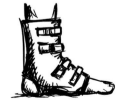

If so, what drives the inflammation? What about hyperinsulinemia (excess insulin)? Because of the complex system that comprises the human body, we have to look at issues like gout from all angles.

Fructose is a vital component of table sugar, making up 50 percent of the sucrose molecule; the other 50 percent is glucose. We've seen that as fructose consumption goes up, the incidence of gout also goes up. Coincidentally, markers of inflammation and uric acid levels also rise as fructose consumption increases. Alcohol is another major contributor to higher uric acid levels. Like fructose, higher alcohol consumption tends to increase the incidence of gout.

One caveat is that if someone already has gout or is strongly predisposed to it, that person may experience a flare up during the transition phase into a ketogenic or carnivore diet. The flare-up is likely a result of a preexisting inflamed state combined with entering into a state of nutritional ketosis, or it's because a transient uric acid elevation is a likely reason for the short-term occurrence of gout. After a person has fully transitioned to an all-meat diet, the gout generally subsides for good.

What About Cancer?

Some researchers have said that red meat leads to colon cancer. In 2015, the World Health Organization (WHO) proclaimed that red meat was a class 2 carcinogen and that processed meat was a class 1 carcinogen, which puts it in the same category as smoking cigarettes in terms of the risk of developing colon cancer. The level of relative risk was around 17 percent for red meat and 18 percent for processed meat.

Scientists from all over the world have criticized this proclamation for several reasons. Independent observers of the process that the International Agency for Research on Cancer (IARC) used to inform the WHO's declaration have pointed out that it was not a consensus decision because approximately 30 percent of the participants disagreed. About 800 studies were considered, but only about 50 were deemed worthy of supporting the position that meat causes cancer; the other studies were thrown out for various reasons.

Dr. Georgia Ede has done a remarkable job of sorting through the same data that the IARC cited, and she's determined that the evidence in support of the claim that meat causes cancer appears to be fairly underwhelming. You can find Dr. Ede's critique at DiagnosisDiet.com, and it's well worth reading. To summarize, her findings show that the vast majority of the data comes from epidemiology, which always lumps true meat eaters with those people who eat junk like burgers, shakes, and fries. Much of the other research was based on rat studies in which the animals were genetically bred to develop cancer, given a cancer-inducing drug, and then fed meat and some toxic rat chow. These types of studies are hardly applicable to a normal human being who eats a healthy diet that includes meat, and the studies in no way accurately represent the habits of a purely carnivorous human. Among those studies on rats and mice were a majority that didn't support the hypothesis that meat causes cancer, and there even exists a study that concludes that bacon was relatively protective against colon cancer. Dr. David Klurfeld, who was one of the IARC panel members, has recently spoken out about the process. He was fairly concerned that contradictory evidence was dismissed and that a large percentage of the panelists were vegan or vegetarian but did not disclose that information on the review.

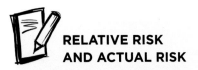

RELATIVE RISK AND ACTUAL RISK

I'll use an example to put relative risk and actual risk in perspective. If the odds that a person will be struck by lightning go from one in one million to two in one million as height increases, the *relative risk* has doubled (increased by 100%), and that sounds kind of scary. However, if we look at the increase in *actual risk*, the difference is only greater by one more in one million, or 0.00001 percent, which is not so scary.

Let's assume that the weak evidence that the WHO used was sufficient to suggest a true relative risk increase in cancer of 18 percent. What does that mean? Well, the generally accepted lifetime risk of developing colon cancer is about 4 percent. If the WHO is correct, that risk goes to 5 percent. In other words, based on the data that supports the WHO's claim, there's a whopping 1 percent increase in absolute risk. This is one of the classic statistical numbers games used to scare people from consuming something that someone doesn't like for various reasons. As always, meat consumption is not the only factor in the risk of developing cancer; we also could look at things like hyperinsulinemia, abdominal obesity, and chronic inflammation (and we could paint a far scarier picture).

As I see it, there are two possible approaches to the WHO's decree: You can question the findings of the WHO because of the poor science backing them, or you can put the findings in context with other factors to determine your overall risk. People who follow a carnivore diet often report greatly improved insulin status, lower levels of abdominal obesity, and significantly reduced inflammation. When you put the whole package together, you find that overall risk for colon cancer likely falls for people on a carnivore diet. Remember—when we talk about associational data, you always should ask, "Does this apply to all people in all situations?" Rats that have been genetically bred to develop cancer and have been given a drug that promotes cancer shouldn't chase down a bolus of toxic rat chow with a steak . Similarly, people who spend their lives eating sugar, vegetable oils, and refined grains and become insulin resistant and obese may want to avoid triple bacon burgers with a side of fries and a shake.

What About Maintaining Proper Nutrition?

The end goal of nutrition has a simple two-pronged explanation: It provides us with energy, and it gives us structural components to build and maintain our animal-based cells. We don't need anything from a plant to accomplish either of those goals. Anything your animal cells need is found in other animal cells. It's as simple as that. You don't need a bunch of indigestible plant fiber or chlorophyll. Plant antioxidants, which we can barely absorb, aren't necessary, either. You only need animal cells—that's it! The nutrients that your animal cells use are also in the cells of other animals that use those same nutrients. How much you need varies only by amount, not by quality. Shockingly, you can get the correct amount of the nutrients because you have something called an *appetite* that lets you know when you need to eat more. It's as simple as that, and every other animal on the planet uses the same feedback system.

But we humans have developed things like the Recommended Daily Allowances, and an army of dietitians teaches us how to meet those magic numbers even though they were formulated from what was just a guess. I will keep reiterating one point: *Nutrition science is based around fundamental assumptions that have never been thoroughly tested.* The carnivore diet is directly challenging some of those untested assumptions, so we're getting new evidence about those theories all the time.

For example, let's look at how the carnivore diet is challenging the assumptions about antioxidants. We're always being encouraged to eat foods that are high in antioxidants, but did you know that they're formed endogenously by the human body. The antioxidants that our bodies produce work extremely well for humans. Plants also produce antioxidants, which work well for plants. You may be surprised to learn that plant antioxidants are basically worthless in terms of the function of the human body. That's right. All the money we've spent over the years to pay for the latest super berry–infused wonder food has been a big waste of money! In fact, some studies indicate that plant antioxidants are potentially harmful to humans. Other studies have shown that we upregulate our endogenous production of antioxidants as we adopt low-carbohydrate diets, so if we want more antioxidants, all we have to do is eat fewer carbs or even exercise.

One of the most disturbing bits of propaganda about eating meat is that it results in a shortened life span. This fallacy is widely pushed by vegan advocates who have a strong penchant for distorting science or cherry-picking studies to support their ethically based beliefs. They almost invariably quote some epidemiologic study that clearly cannot prove anything beyond a weak association. Among their favorites are the studies that come from Loma Linda University and the Adventist health system, whose foundations are linked inextricably to a religious philosophy that promotes vegetarianism. Possible bias or conflict of interest? I say, "Heck, yeah!" We can easily find several recent studies that show no difference in life span between people who avoid meat and people who enjoy it.

We can look at two populations and find two very different outcomes. The two groups include the historical Inuit, who were largely free of disease but had a life span shorter than their nonindigenous neighbors and the citizens of the city-state of Hong Kong, who eat (by far) the most meat of any major population center in the world and are among the longest-lived people on the planet. The Inuit live in abject poverty and crowded conditions, and they have high smoking rates, which are two contributors to shorter life spans. Conversely, citizens of Hong Kong live in an area of tremendous wealth and security. The long life spans of Hong Kong residents don't prove that meat makes people have longevity, but it definitely makes it hard to say that meat shortens one's life span. The lesson here is that wealth leads to a long life; poverty, not meat, shortens it.

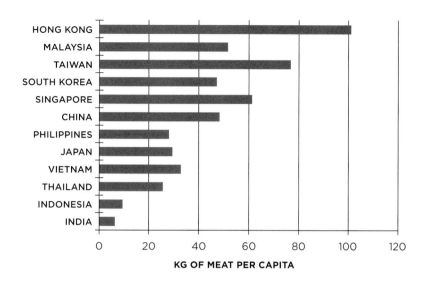

Highest Longevity Rates (in Years)

Women		Men	
Hong Kong	87.66	Hong Kong	81.70
Japan	87.26	Switzerland	81.5
Spain	85.84	Japan	81.09
South Korea	85.4	Norway	80.91
France, Switzerland	85.3	Sweden	80.72

Figure 4.2 (source: Japanese Ministry of Health, Labour, and Welfare)

Could it be that a meat-based diet results in greater longevity or better health span regardless of other factors? Well, we could certainly make that hypothesis based on several observations. We know that carnosine, which is a molecule in plentiful supply in meat, is perhaps the most powerful substance for reducing oxidative stress and preventing the formation of something called advanced glycation end products (AGEs), which are associated with aging. An interesting study published in *Nutrition Journal* in 2016 looked at telomere length and found that red meat was the only food that had a favorable effect on the telomeres. Telomeres are a portion of the ends of our DNA strands that some researchers think are a measure of cellular aging. Also, researchers have identified a relationship between strength and health span and life span. A diet high in animal protein supports maintaining and building strength. In terms of general metabolic health, we again see the effect of insulin on numerous diseases of lifestyle, and through laboratory studies into the regression of disease states, it's becoming clear that all-meat diets are improving insulin function dramatically.

One of the more comical and desperate attempts to dissuade people from eating animals is a recent campaign launched by People for the Ethical Treatment of Animals (PETA) that claimed that eating meat leads to impotence and the ruination of one's sex life. This idea is particularly humorous because, if anything, the exact opposite happens. We can look to the Kellogg brothers at the end of the nineteenth century, who attempted to ban people from eating meat because it was known to lead to lustful behavior. What was true back then remains so today; I see a continuous stream of men and women who report having supercharged libido and sexual function after adopting a carnivore diet. This fallacy once again ties to the worthless epidemiology in which the "burger, shakes, and fries" crowd is conflated to a healthy meat eater. When we look at the junk food eaters who consume the standard American diet, we see vascular problems. And many meat eaters also tend to eat the junk as well as the meat. It's just as simple as that. Eat meat and no junk (like a true carnivore), and things are great. Eat meat plus junk (or, worse, eat only the junk), and things are bad.

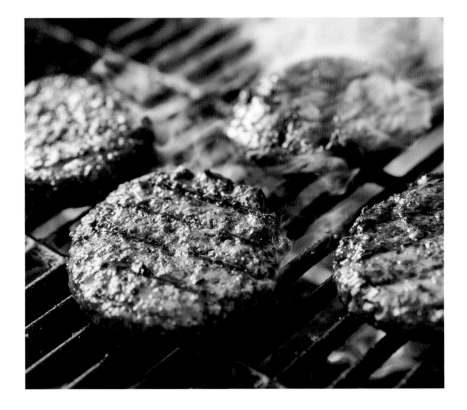

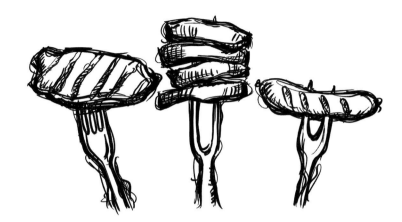

MEAT,
THE SUPERFOOD

Let's talk about meat. Many cultures throughout the world have prized it. Civilizations appeased the gods with burnt offerings of sacrificed animals. Indigenous populations spend hours each day in the quest for meat, despite being surrounded by edible plant food options. Wealth historically has been discussed in terms of cattle owned, and meat was often reserved for the rich, and the lower classes had to make do with a few scraps here and there. In emerging countries like China, which has a population of almost 1.4 billion people, the burgeoning middle class is now demanding meat.

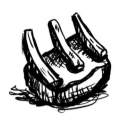

Why is meat such a staple across cultures? Human life demands it. It's one of our most primitive needs. Eating meat is as vital to our survival as breathing. If we don't provide our bodies with a regular supply, then our bodies begin to cannibalize our tissues to make up for the deficit. As some people age, they lose the capacity to chew, and then they subsequently become unable to digest meat properly. That's when the slow reabsorption of body tissues begins, and we start to see issues like sarcopenia, which is the loss of muscle mass. We lose bone mass, which is about 40 percent protein. Our production of vital hormones, neurotransmitters, and basic cell functions starts to fail. Eventually, our very existence becomes one of daily pain, weakness, and despair. We often spend a significant portion of our lives propped up by pills to control symptoms and functional aids to help us navigate daily activities, and we spend vast resources on medical care that's often minimally effective.

People who've adopted all-meat diets often report feeling two or three decades younger. Their chronic pains go away, their desire for life returns, and their diseases resolve or remit. For some people, the changes have been downright miraculous. People who have given up on life and suffer chronic depression have seen profound reversals in their mental states. For the first time in memory, they find that they're happy and looking forward to life. Let's talk about why these changes may happen.

Meat offers a tremendous amount of nutrition, even though it's vilified for having cholesterol and saturated fat (which are vital components of the human body). As I pointed out in an earlier chapter, meat is made of basically the same stuff that we are made of. I know this concept is novel for many people, but let's think about it for a minute and ignore what we "know" based on epidemiology and the highly flawed RDA system. If you want to build a car and you have access to a pile of car parts or a pile of computers, from which one would you draw your supplies? Also, does it make sense to assume that all cells in our bodies require the same essential vitamins, minerals, fats, and amino acids, or is it more likely that liver cells require certain nutrients, whereas muscle cells have a completely different set of requirements? All cells need the same basic stuff. Therefore, if all cells require those nutrients, we can conclude that all cells also contain those nutrients. I don't need to eat specialized cells to feed the cells in my body. I can take all the nutrients from a rib-eye steak, which is made up of a bunch of animal cells, and then turn them into whatever my body needs. This is by far the most efficient way to feed my body provided I eat enough. Yes, we have a limited capacity to turn material from plants into what we need, but the process is much less efficient than drawing nutrients from meat, and it comes with some drawbacks, which I address in the next chapter.

Meat is rich in several unique compounds found exclusively, or almost exclusively, in animal-based foods. These compounds include carnitine, carnosine, creatine, taurine, retinol, and vitamins B12, D3, and K2. These compounds offer some tremendous benefits.

Carnosine

Carnosine is a dipeptide molecule (meaning it has two amino acids) that is tremendously effective at preventing glycation, and it works to scavenge oxygen free radicals. It can chelate (or bind to) metal ions and appears to prevent the shortening of telomeres. Carnosine's antiglycating properties can help mitigate the development of things like Alzheimer's disease, atherosclerosis, and renal disease. Carnosine is taken up in its intact state in the digestive system and is transported via a dipeptide transporter. Muscle levels of carnosine are significantly higher in people who eat meat compared to the levels in their vegetarian counterparts. By some accounts, carnosine may be one of the most potent antiaging molecules known.

> Glycation occurs when a sugar molecule (often glucose or fructose) attaches itself to another structure; it often attaches to proteins but also fats and nucleic acid found in DNA. Once the sugar molecule is attached, it can cause the structure to become distorted and lose its normal strength and function.

Carnitine

Like carnosine, carnitine is found almost exclusively in animal products, especially red meat. In comparisons of meat eaters and nonmeat eaters, carnitine levels are higher in the meat eaters. Carnitine has several potentially beneficial effects in preventing and improving diseases. It has been shown to help with anemia, particularly for anemia associated with kidney dysfunction. It appears to improve the body's use of glucose, and it may reduce the effects of diabetic peripheral neuropathy. In heart attack patients, carnitine has been used to prevent ischemia in cardiac muscle, and it's even been shown to assist with resolving male infertility via an improvement in sperm quality. Additionally, carnitine plays a crucial metabolic role in transporting free fatty acids across the mitochondrial membrane for energy production. Carnitine is a vital component, and we can synthesize it from the amino acid lysine, which we also obtain from eating animal products.

A study published in the journal *Urology* in 2004, in which the effects of carnitine were compared to the effects of testosterone, found that carnitine was superior for promoting better erection capacity than testosterone. Perhaps this is one of the reasons so many men report improved sexual capacity and libido when they follow a carnivore diet.

One concern about carnitine is that certain intestinal bacteria can convert it into a substance called trimethylamine (TMA), which later potentially can be converted to the oxidized form in the liver called trimethylamine N-oxide (TMAO). In animal studies, TMAO has been associated with higher rates of atherosclerosis, and one study observed that humans with high levels have an increased risk of cardiac disease. Some critics of this study, including Dr. Georgia Ede, contend that the genetically altered mice were fed a supplementary form of carnitine that's not in meat, and the people with higher TMAO levels had unknown diets. So basically, we have no idea whether meat eaters, and especially carnivore dieters, have abnormally high levels of TMAO or whether TMAO has a causative role or is an associational bystander. Also, fish and vegetables, which traditionally have been viewed as being "good" foods, also have been shown to cause a rise in TMAO levels, which is something that undermines the whole "meat is bad because of TMAO" argument.

Creatine

Creatine, a supplement athletes commonly use and one of the few that's been found to be beneficial after being rigorously tested, is another product found only in meat. Meat eaters register higher levels of creatine, and when vegetarians supplement creatine, they experience improved cognitive function. It's also interesting to note that patients with Alzheimer's disease have lower levels of creatine. Heart failure patients who receive creatine have shown improved overall performance, and type 2 diabetics who supplement with creatine have improved glycemic control, particularly when they also exercise.

Taurine

Taurine is found in high levels in both meat and fish but is woefully absent from a plant-based diet. As you might expect, taurine levels are significantly lower among herbivorous humans. In animal studies, taurine has been shown to reduce anxiety. Perhaps that is one reason so many folks on a carnivore diet report a sense of calmness and a resolution of anxiety.

Taurine is similar to carnosine and has been shown to inhibit glycation. It's also a powerful antioxidant. Some evidence suggests that taurine contributes to preventing the development of diabetic renal disease.

Zinc

Although zinc is not exclusive to animal products, it's found in much greater quantity and is more highly bioavailable in meat, and numerous plants containing phytates interfere with zinc's absorption. Accordingly, zinc levels are fairly low in vegan and vegetarian dieters. Zinc deficiency has been associated with poor learning capacity, apathy, and behavioral problems in children. In adult males, low levels of zinc are associated with erectile dysfunction and decreased sperm counts. Zinc also is essential in the formation of insulin and has been shown to improve glycemic control among some diabetics. Zinc appears to have a protective effect in preventing coronary artery disease and cardiomyopathy. Zinc is involved in a whole bunch of metabolic processes throughout the body, and being deficient in zinc is not a good thing.

Vitamin B12

Vitamin B12, also known as cobalamin, is found exclusively in animal products, and experts advise people who abstain from meat to supplement it. One of the more common causes of deficiency is gastrointestinal malabsorption. Up to 62 percent of pregnant vegan women were noted to be deficient in B12, and up to 86 percent of vegan children and 90 percent of vegan elderly were B12-deficient. B12 deficiency typically affects the nervous system and can cause problems with anemia. A deficit of vitamin B12 has been associated with several neurological diseases, including dementia; it's also related to depression. I know eating a big juicy steak always makes me happy. Maybe it's from all the B12 I'm getting!

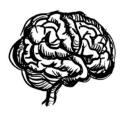

Heme Iron

Heme iron is another mineral found in abundance in red meat but absent from nonmeat sources. Unsurprisingly, a 2015 study of vegetarian women saw a 100 percent rate of some degree of iron deficiency anemia, which was more than double the rate of deficiency in their omnivorous counterparts. Certain plants, like leafy greens, soybeans, and lentils, contain non-heme iron, but those plants also can contain compounds like phytates and oxalates that limit iron absorption. The functions of iron are multiple; some of the highlights are the formation of red blood cells, transport of oxygen, support of immune function, support of cognition, and assistance with energy metabolism.

Deficiency of iron has been shown to result in impairments in cognition and mental health status and a sense of general fatigue. Those symptoms have been shown to improve with supplementation. Low iron status has been associated with worsening glycemic control and has been shown to be a factor that increases the risk for several types of cancer, such as pancreatic and kidney cancer. Conversely, excessive iron stores, which is a far less frequent situation, can be associated with several negative outcome measures. Inflammation and metabolic syndrome seem to predispose people to iron overload, and these conditions are frequently associated with each other. Thus far, most anecdotal observations of strict carnivores show that their inflammatory markers are typically very low, their metabolic markers are very favorable, and their iron statuses generally are in the normal range, despite their ingestion of large amounts of heme iron.

On average, people who include meat in their diets generally have better vitamin and mineral status than those who do not, and the vast majority of nutritional deficiency problems are in parts of the world where access to meat is scarce. In impoverished locations where meat is abundant, it's not common to see nutritional deficiencies, whereas in poorer areas where people rely on a plant-based diet, residents frequently suffer from stunted growth and have numerous nutritional deficiency syndromes.

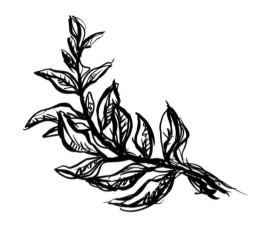

CHAPTER SIX

THE MYTH OF PLANTY GOODNESS

The belief that fruits and vegetables are good for us is based on faith more than it's based on science. We've all been told by our parents to eat our vegetables because they're good for us. Questioning that parental advice is deeply troubling for most people. Why would our parents force us to eat vegetables if they weren't making us healthy? Many of us remember that Popeye used to chug cans of spinach to get super strength before going to battle against his nemesis, Bluto, which only lent more weight to our parents' position on vegetables.

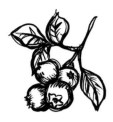

Plants have been on the planet for roughly 700 million years, and they have been successfully fighting off various fungi, insects, and other animals since well before humans arrived some 3 million years ago. Plants have developed all kinds of defense strategies to ensure the survival of their species, including a system of elaborate chemical defenses. If you and I (or perhaps our ancestor, good ol' Urk) were to go walking in the wilderness, and we started eating random plants, we would very quickly find ourselves either very sick or dead. Of the approximately 400,000 species of plants on Earth, only a tiny fraction are edible by humans. Among the edible plants, typically only a portion of the plant is safe to eat; the rest is often harmful to humans. Even today, plant poisonings are still relatively common events.

Most of the produce that we see in the supermarket has absolutely no resemblance whatsoever to the plants that would have been available to Urk and his peers 50,000 years ago. Cruciferous vegetables basically didn't exist, and Urk would have avoided leafy greens because of their extremely bitter taste. Tubers and other starchy "underground storage organs" were not particularly tasty and would have been primarily composed of fibrous, tough material. Nuts and seeds are well-protected physically by a tough outer shell or more subtly by toxic chemical defenses. Unprocessed nuts or beans can be among the most deadly plant-based foods around. Plants are especially protective of their offspring. The fruits we eat today have been manipulated to the point that prehistoric Urk wouldn't recognize them.

As the megafaunal animals began to die off, starting around 25,000 or so years ago, humans became increasingly dependent upon getting energy from smaller, less fatty animals. They needed other ways to supplement that energy, so humans learned how to exploit a progressively greater number of plants. Fruits, nuts, and seeds, which would have provided the most bang for the buck calorically, were likely some of the early go-to plants. Our ancestors probably worked through thousands of generations of careful experimentation to separate plants into the "that'll kill ya," the "you'll get a little bit sick," and the "seems okay to me and doesn't taste too bad" categories.

As time passed, more people ate these foods with greater frequency and increasing volume; eventually, agriculture and the domestication of grain resulted in a wholesale shift in nutrition and made the development of more stabilized communities possible. The nomadic or pastoral lifestyle started to be replaced by villages, towns, and cities. During this time when plants were being hybridized, cultivated, and otherwise processed to become more edible, randomized controlled trials weren't being conducted to determine their long-term safety. If no one got acutely ill, that plant was deemed acceptable to use as food.

We know that plants are full of chemicals, many of which serve as pesticides. If we had to introduce those same natural plant pesticides to the market today and subject them to rigorous toxicity testing, many of those chemicals would not be allowed on the market. However, because there is no real regulatory organization that examines "natural substances" in food, we tend not to worry about it.

I'm not saying that researchers have never studied these naturally occurring plant compounds in everyday fruits and vegetables. In fact, there are numerous studies on this topic. In 1990, famed toxicology researcher Professor Bruce Ames investigated the use of pesticides in food production and compared manufactured pesticides to naturally occurring plant-chemical pesticides. Shockingly, Ames found that 99.9 percent of pesticides we consume by volume comes from plants themselves. When he examined some of these compounds in more detail, a majority were shown to cause cancer in animal models. We shouldn't run away from all fruits and vegetables because of a potential cancer risk. However, it does show us that there are plenty of chemicals in the plant foods we eat, and many of them have a potentially negative effect. The potential risk consideration of plants' defensive chemicals is outside the more commonly accepted risks associated with excess sugar, refined grains, and seed oils, which more and more people are coming to accept as problematic. As we observe a growing number of people who experience dramatic improvement in things like autoimmune diseases, mental health disorders, and chronic gastrointestinal diseases when they completely remove plants from their diets, it becomes fairly easy to wonder whether some of the potentially noxious chemicals in plants may have a role in our problems even at low-dose chronic exposure. Because we rarely (if ever) test for those types of effects, we may have to wait a long time to find answers to those questions. Meanwhile, we have an ever-growing list of so-called "idiopathic diseases," which basically means we have no clue what's causing the problem, so we blame it on bad luck, genetics, or perhaps stress.

To be fair, researchers have done quite a few epidemiologic studies that indicate that eating more fruits, vegetables, and fiber is associated with favorable population health outcomes. There are even some interventional trials that indicate the same thing. Is there any truth to that? Certainly, but it doesn't answer the question we're asking, which is whether plant-based foods are inherently good and necessary. When you examine the studies, the researchers always have evaluated a mixed diet, often the standard American diet, so they've looked at the effects of adding fruits and vegetables to the other garbage many people eat. Sure, if the result is that you eat less sugary, oily, processed garbage because you're eating more fruits and vegetables, then you would expect to see a benefit. Do any studies compare an all-meat or meat-based diet to a more plant-based diet? Nope, no one

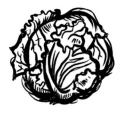

has ever done that. So all we can assume is that eating fruits and vegetables is better than eating a mixed diet that includes donuts and potato chips. Wow, what a revelation! Glad my tax dollars went there.

Plants Waging Chemical Warfare

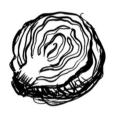

The list of chemicals found in the plants we commonly consume is extensive, and I'm not going to list them all. However, I'm covering some of the more common ones so I can talk about the potential and documented effects. Remember, researchers have studied many of these compounds in limited capacities, and we likely will never know all the potential interactions and issues that may be related to them. It's also important to note that although a particular compound may cause a major problem in one person, another person may not experience any obvious issues.

Oxalates

Commonly found in leafy green vegetables, some fruits, nuts, seeds, and even French fries, oxalates are a pretty common antinutrient. They can lead to medical problems—particularly when people ingest them in higher doses. One of the most common issues is kidney stones, which often are comprised of oxalates. Oxalate crystals in the body can become very needlelike, and some research has associated them with gastrointestinal irritation. The crystals may lead to leaky gut syndrome and potentially can lead to autoimmune issues. Interestingly, oxalates are often in foods we find on typical ketogenic diets (for example, leafy greens, almond flour, and dark chocolate). When you stop eating those foods all at once, sometimes you can experience oxalate dumping syndrome, which can manifest in several ways, including rashes, joint pain, and gastrointestinal disturbance.

Lectins

Lectins, recently made popular by Dr. Steven Gundry's book, *The Plant Paradox*, are a fairly ubiquitous plant compound, but they're particularly concentrated in things like grains, nuts, corn, quinoa, fruits, nightshades, vegetable oils, legumes, beans, and squash. The trouble with lectins is that they can lead to a leaky gut situation and likely contribute to all the potential downstream effects of leaky gut.

Glycoalkaloids

Glycoalkaloids are in nightshade plants like potatoes, tomatoes, eggplants, and peppers. Limited evidence suggests these compounds have a connection to leaky gut syndrome and autoimmune problems like psoriasis. The foods that contain glycoalkaloids—particularly the nightshade vegetables—have been reported to worsen symptoms of irritable bowel syndrome (IBS).

Goitrogens

Goitrogens are substances that can interfere with the function of the thyroid. Thyroid dysfunction is particularly common among women, and some researchers believe that high amounts of goitrogen-containing foods may play a role. Foods like soy and cruciferous vegetables tend to be high in these substances. Perhaps all those years of forcing ourselves to choke down broccoli and cauliflower were not kind to our thyroids.

Cyanogenic Glycosides

Cyanogenic glycosides are in common foods like almonds, flaxseed, linseed, lima beans, cassava, and certain stone fruits (such as cherries, peaches, and plums). Cyanide poisonings can and do occur, commonly with consumption of cassava root; sometimes death is the result of poisoning. Chronic exposure to cyanides is postulated to contribute to chronic diseases such as impaired thyroid function and neurological disturbances.

Phytic Acid

Phytic acid is in grains, seeds, nuts, and legumes. It can lead to mineral deficiencies, particularly deficiency of zinc, calcium, magnesium, and iron. Deficiencies in these minerals can lead to a host of potential problems, including heart disease, depression, infertility, impotence, hair loss, and compromised immune function. On the beneficial side, phytic acid has been shown to lower blood glucose and potentially lessen the formation of kidney stones.

Protease Inhibitors

Protease inhibitors are in most legumes, particularly soy; cereals; fruits such as kiwi, pineapple, papaya, bananas, figs, and apples; and vegetables such as cabbage, potatoes, tomatoes, and cucumbers. The protease inhibitors interfere with the activity of enzymes involved with protein digestion, such as trypsin, and in animal studies, they have been shown to lead to poor growth in subjects. Conversely, there is some evidence to show these compounds may have a positive role in limiting cancer.

Flavonoids

Flavonoids, which are responsible for some of the pigment found in plants, are commonly found in citrus fruit, cocoa, blueberries, parsley, onions, and bananas. They're potentially beneficial at low levels, but in higher doses, they've been noted to cause genetic mutations, oxidation that leads to free radical production, and inhibition of hormones.

Saponins

Saponins are in legumes, beans, garlic, alfalfa sprouts, peas, yucca, and asparagus. They have been shown to cause digestive disturbances, thyroid problems, and damage to red blood cells. Fun stuff indeed!

Salicylates

Salicylates are in many fruits and vegetables and some spices. They're often responsible for sensitivity reactions that can trigger asthma, gut inflammation, and diarrhea.

Plants' Presumed Innocence

There are easily dozens of other chemical compounds in plants, and it's all the same song and dance. A plant makes a chemical; the chemical causes problems in some cases but in other cases has a beneficial effect. In studies of the chemicals, we often see a confirmation bias to support the epidemiology (and what our parents have always told us) about the benefits of vegetables and fruits. I've read countless studies on this stuff, and it's almost comical to see that nearly every paper starts with, "We all know that people who eat fruits and vegetables are healthy." Then the author goes on to describe a study on some isolated plant compound that shows why fruits and vegetables are good for us. These researchers aren't testing a hypothesis; they're merely trying to confirm it. Hence we have reports that cruciferous vegetables prevent cancer, even though we have data to show that it can either increase *or* decrease the occurrence of cancer. However, because the existing epidemiology says cruciferous vegetables *prevent* cancer, we favor the positive data and tend to ignore the negative data.

If I believed that drinking gasoline was a good thing, perhaps because my grandfather told me it was a good thing, and we also conducted a small epidemiologic study that showed that people who've ingested gasoline had less incidence of cancer-related death, I'm sure I could design another study to support that conclusion. For example, I could easily take cultured cancer cells and then expose them to various doses of gasoline until I found one that inhibited the growth of cancer cells. Voilà—we now have a mechanistic method by which to show gasoline drinking is healthy and may lower rates of cancer. These situations abound in the literature. Someone looks at an isolated compound in an isolated scenario, which is then extrapolated to the whole of human physiology to support an epidemiologic claim.

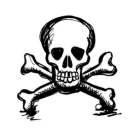

There is a small number of studies that look at whole plant foods and their effects on the human physiology or disease process. Once again, I credit Dr. Georgia Ede for working hard to dig through the literature on this topic and summarizing it in her article about vegetables at her website, Diagnosis: Diet. There are about two dozen studies that look at actual trials on humans in which fruits or vegetables in their whole form were examined rather than an isolated plant compound being investigated in an epidemiologic or animal/cell culture study. The overall result of these studies is that whole fruits and vegetables show only limited or no significant benefit. In some cases, the effects are slightly deleterious, with vegetables being worse than fruits.

Nutrition science continues to make the same mistakes over and over again; we rely heavily on epidemiology and then merely try to use further study to confirm the findings rather than refute them. If you look at an epidemiologic study that shows people who eat more fruits and vegetables appear healthy, you easily could conclude that eating plant-based foods is a healthy thing to do. That's a very logical conclusion, and no one would fault you for making it. However, if you ask some different questions, things get more interesting. Let's say that people who eat fruits and vegetables avoid eating snack cakes, donuts, and sodas. Perhaps they smoke less, drink less alcohol, wear their seat belt, exercise more, have more wealth, and can live in a nicer area. All these things, and likely dozens of other things, contribute to what is known as the "healthy user bias." In other words, if your overall lifestyle tends to be healthful, how much of the observed improvements in health outcome is attributable to the other factors versus the one particular food being studied. The epidemiologist will attempt to control for these other factors, but really she's just guessing how much each factor contributes.

I've already mentioned some glaring examples of situations where the epidemiology suggests one thing, but real life suggests another. For example, meat is supposedly bad for us and will shorten our lives, yet the population of Hong Kong eats more meat than any other population in the world, and they also live the longest. This observation sets off the immediate cries of, "But they don't smoke as much; they're wealthy; they exercise," and so on, and it's fine that people make those arguments. However, when we make the same argument that fruits and vegetables are bad for us, we tend to hear silence from those same people. Nutrition is like politics, and people fight hard for their team. Results that don't confirm a particular bias are quickly ignored or dismissed. Questioning the current dogma often is met with anger and an almost religious deference to authority and the "consensus"; however, those questions that challenge the status quo should be embraced in a true scientific community.

It's heretical to suggest that fruits and vegetables are anything but goodness, rainbows, and unicorns. Yeah, we acknowledge that they may have chemicals in them that can cause issues, but, by golly, we still say you need to eat your five (no wait, it's now ten) servings per day.

ICELAND

Iceland, a frozen island of fearsome Vikings, has a population of only about 300,000 people. They've historically relied heavily on an animal-based diet because fruits and vegetables just don't grow in that climate. Iceland has produced nine winners of the World's Strongest Man contest. The only other country with more winners is the United States, which boasts eleven champions and a population 1,000 times as big as Iceland. Icelandic women have won four of the twelve CrossFit titles as well. Despite traditionally having little access to fruits and vegetables, Iceland is among the world's leaders in male centenarians per capita. What does Iceland's production of strong people and centenarians say about our belief that you have to have a certain number of vegetables and fruits per day to be healthy?

Quick, tell me which fruit, vegetable, or other plant is an absolutely essential requirement for human life? If you can think of one, then I'd like to know whether it grows all year round and in all parts of the world. If we have essential requirements for them—and we don't—we would have had limited access to them for roughly 99 percent of our time on Earth as a species. Given that, why does it make sense to recommend we eat copious amounts of fruits and vegetables every day?

Humans survived an Ice Age, which means our ancestors' habitat was like Iceland, not Costa Rica. If we're willing to set aside our arrogance about how much we think we know and apply some commonsense observations, we can see how impractical a diet full of indigestible fiber and nonessential phytonutrients is. We need fat, protein, and some vitamins and minerals. We require no other nutrients to live or—I'll argue—to thrive. We require zero carbohydrates, zero phytochemicals, and zero fiber.

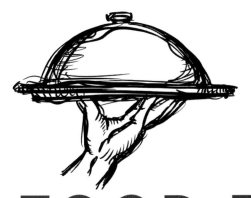

CHAPTER SEVEN

LET FOOD BE THY MEDICINE AND OTHER HERESY

At this point, it should be clear that I believe nutrition plays a tremendous role in the development, prevention, and mitigation of darn near every common chronic disease. If nutrition affects disease, as I believe it does, then what happens when hundreds of thousands of people try to use a select nutritional scheme to fix a chronic issue. Well, certainly there will be a ton of noise created in the medical community, and there will be an endless supply of bias and plenty of confusing data. Sounds kind of like the system we have in place. Eventually, though, I believe that some signal will rise above the noise, and the cream will rise to the top. People will cast aside that which does not work and will replace it with that which does.

In this chapter, I discuss some of the medical conditions that I have found to respond favorably to a meat-based diet. For some reason, we seem to think that the presence of a disease automatically means we need some pharmaceutical and that it's impossible for something as lowly as food to contribute to many of our diseases. I am continually impressed by the ever-growing list of conditions that we discover are alleviated by a change in diet. These are often idiopathic (we don't have a clue what causes them) or autoimmune disorders. Amazingly, even some genetic disorders are relieved by dietary changes.

The Carnivore Diet and Chronic Disease

I know from years of taking care of patients that most chronic diseases don't go away; instead, they slowly worsen with time. I also admit that I am biased, as is every other human on the planet. I firmly believe that eating a meat-based diet can help alleviate issues caused by chronic diseases. I've had the good fortune to have thousands of people who've shared their stories of their experiences with pursuing a carnivore diet. The stuff they tell me has shocked me—in a good way. People have told me of a plethora of conditions that have either completely resolved or significantly improved when they've followed a carnivore diet. Here's a sample:

ADHD	Bipolar disorder	Dental caries
Alcohol dependence	Boils	Depression
Amenorrhea	Bulimia	Dermatofibroma
Anemia	Candidiasis	Diabetes mellitus
Angina	Carpal tunnel syndrome	Diverticulitis
Ankylosing spondylitis	Cholelithiasis	Diverticulosis
Anxiety	Chronic bronchitis	Dupuytren's contracture
Arthritis	Chronic fatigue syndrome	Eczema
Asthma	COPD	Ehlers-Danlos syndrome
Athlete's foot	Cocaine dependence	Epicondylitis
Atopic dermatitis	Colitis	Epilepsy
Autism	Crohn's disease	Erectile dysfunction

Fatty liver	Irritable bowel syndrome	Rosacea
Fibromyalgia	Juvenile rheumatoid arthritis	Sciatica
Floaters	Keloids	Scleroderma
Gerd	Lipoma	Synovitis
Gingivitis	Lyme disease	Systemic lupus erythematosus
Gout	Meniere's disease	Tinnitus
Hashimoto's thyroiditis	Narcolepsy	Trichotillomania
Headache/migraine	Nephrolithiasis	Trigger finger
Hemorrhoids	Neuropathy	Ulcerative colitis
Hidradenitis suppurativa	Parkinson's disease	
Hypertension	PCOS	
Hypertriglyceridemia	Psoriasis/psoriatic arthritis	
Hypothyroidism	Quadriceps tendonitis	
Insulin resistance	Rheumatoid arthritis	

I could go on and on with the list, but I wanted to give you just a taste of all the ailments that seem to respond positively to the carnivore diet. To be clear, I'm talking about anecdotal reports of people who've self-reported their progress, and I acknowledge that there are several problems with anecdotal data like this. (And critics of this type of data are in no short supply.) People provide anecdotal reports about all sorts of things, such as that they've seen UFOs or that the Virgin Mary has spoken to them via a piece of wood. They report that they've seen Bigfoot and the Yeti, or that they've had their cancer cured by witchcraft. However, the fact that some anecdotes seem outlandish doesn't mean that all are completely worthless, and most theory starts with an anecdote or an observation that someone decides to research with a well-planned study.

Let's look at an example of the typical path that a chronic issue follows. Knee pain is a good one. A person might start with some mild knee irritation that occurs after a particular event or activity. With some rest and maybe a few anti-inflammatories, the problem goes away. A few years later, though, the pain is back and becoming a daily problem. Perhaps the doctor prescribes some therapy and suggests trying a longer course of medications. The pain becomes manageable again, but it never really goes away; it's still hanging around in the background. A decade later, the pain becomes very limiting; the knee begins to swell, and stiffness starts to become more and more common. Imaging might reveal some damaged cartilage and perhaps a torn bit of the meniscus. Now the doctor suggests an arthroscopic surgery to "clean up things," although the benefits of such a surgery often are minimal. The patient receives a few months of relief, but the knee continues to ache, swell, and be limiting to the person's activities. Sometimes the doctor administers cortisone or viscosupplementation shots. Like the other treatments, the shots provide minimal to no help as a long-term solution. The patient is basically waiting until the knee gets so bad that replacing the joint is the best solution. Some folks with bad knees put their faith in a stem cell injection or a platelet-rich plasma (PRP) injection. These types of treatments often promise the moon based on the latest science, but they don't deliver on the promise. Even after the knee is replaced, most people continue to experience chronic pain in the knee, albeit at a lower level than before the surgery.

Why do all those treatments result in such a poor outcome? Arthritis is as much a biological inflammatory condition as it is a mechanical phenomenon. When you don't address the biological part, fixing the mechanical part is like installing new carpeting for your floors while your house is on fire. You have to address the inflammatory condition to see long-term relief. I've seen countless people who've essentially resolved their arthritic pain by adopting a carnivore diet, and it often happens within weeks of making the dietary change. I've even known of people who've canceled joint replacement surgeries because their joints had completely stopped hurting. According to conventional medical science, that's not what's supposed to happen. These results are highly unusual, and, if you're like me, you should raise a skeptical eyebrow.

That's exactly what I did. I began to track and consolidate these "miracles." I partnered with a like-minded individual named Matt Maier, and we started organizing this data through a small online endeavor. In 2017, we had several hundred people participate in what we called an N Equals Many project, which was informal but still a bit more structured than collecting some random anecdotes. Of the several hundred people who completed ninety days of a carnivore diet, we found across-the-board improvements in self-reported joint health, gut health, sexual health, mood, skin health, energy, and exercise capacity. We saw an average weight loss of about 30 pounds, waist circumference reduction of 3 inches, and a resting heart rate that was 8 points lower than it had been at the start of the trial. I acknowledge that there are all kinds of potential issues with this type of "study," and I fully recognize the limitations. Still, studies like this give us a starting point to lead to more studies as interest in this subject grows.

I'm not the only one who is beginning to look into the relationship between a fully animal-sourced diet and the resolution of disease. Dr. Csaba Toth is a clinician with a small medical group in Hungary, where they have treated several thousand patients using what they call a paleolithic ketogenic diet. Basically, this diet is purely animal-based; it includes meat with relatively high percentages of fats and some occasional organ meat.

I recently spoke with Dr. Toth, and he told me about the work he and his colleagues are doing to address diet and intestinal permeability. They use a substance called polyethylene glycol to determine a patient's intestinal permeability. When our intestinal permeability is high, we're susceptible to developing what we call a "leaky gut," which is an issue that's now thought to be involved in a number of disease states. Leaky gut and autoimmune problems are highly correlated. Dr. Toth has found that changing the components of the diet markedly affects the intestinal permeability, and the most problematic things we ingest are plant oils, medications, and supplements. The second most problematic group includes grains, legumes, nightshade plants, dairy, and sweeteners. Dr. Toth has found that when a person is on a meat-based diet, the intestinal permeability completely normalizes, markers of inflammation (such as tumor necrosis factor [TNF] alpha and interleukin 6 [IL-6]) declines, and autoimmune symptoms begin to resolve. Among the many conditions that Dr. Toth's practice successfully treats are Crohn's disease, ulcerative colitis, irritable bowel syndrome (IBS), Hashimoto's thyroiditis, type 1 and type 2 diabetes, scleroderma, and systemic lupus erythematosus (SLE). They have several case reports in the literature, and many of the clinic's patients are physicians themselves.

Risk factors for common diseases that are universally problematic include things like obesity (especially abdominal or visceral obesity), hypertension, inflammation, and hyperinsulinemia. The issues are considered risk factors with just about every chronic disease that I can think of. I'm unaware of any situations in which excess belly fat is a good thing. Unlike many lab markers of disease (such as elevated cholesterol) that have to be considered in context, things like belly fat and poor insulin sensitivity are bad regardless of context.

One of the most striking patterns that I see when people embark upon a carnivore diet is a reduction in blood pressure, insulin resistance, inflammation, and body fat. In general, improving all these factors reduces your risk for almost any disease. Heart disease? Yep. Cancer? Yep. Dementia? Yep. Depression? Yep. The list goes on and on. There are all kinds of wailing and gnashing of teeth about how eating red meat raises your absolute risk of colon cancer by one percent (from 4 percent to 5 percent). But if you look at the data on the effects of reducing your abdominal obesity or improving your insulin sensitivity, you can start to put things in perspective with the big picture. In a nutshell, reducing abdominal fat improves almost every single chronic disease we know of. Remember, nothing acts in isolation; you have to consider the whole package. As I've said before, when interpreting large-scale population data associations, you need to ask whether the association holds up for all people in all situations. Almost every single bit of health and nutritional data we've obtained over the last century comes from looking at populations of people who consume the majority

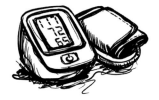

of their calories from a carbohydrate-laden diet. Are the normal reference ranges applicable to someone on a low-carbohydrate diet or a carnivore diet? The answer is that we just don't know because those studies haven't been done yet.

We certainly shouldn't accept "We just don't know" as a final answer. Fortunately, we're starting to see some common patterns emerging as more and more people get comfortable in the low-carb, ketogenic, and carnivore space. We often see elevations in total and LDL cholesterol; that pattern is often accompanied by low levels of triglycerides, favorable triglyceride/HDL ratios, good insulin status, low blood pressure, and low levels of inflammation. Should we consider this a normal variant, or should we still go running scared and start pounding the statin drugs to bring down the total and LDL cholesterol numbers? Many people are starting to challenge the widely held belief that high cholesterol leads to heart disease, and we're now starting to see examples of people who live in a constant state of higher-than-normal cholesterol but whose arteries are perfectly clean when they're examined. I recently had my coronary arteries tested with something called a coronary artery calcium scan, which many believe is one of the best tests to determine cardiac risk. My score was a perfect zero even though I've had elevated LDL and total cholesterol for many years and have been eating an average of four pounds of red meat per day for several years. Again, this phenomenon of high cholesterol with an absence of cardiovascular disease merits further study and long-term follow-up, but until people actually test it, the long-term data will never come.

Does it seem scary that some people roll the dice to be guinea pigs by trying the carnivore diet without having research to back up the claims? I would argue that most of Western society have been involuntary guinea pigs in a giant, failed low-fat experiment that has left us fatter and sicker than at any other point in our existence! We could even make the argument that the introduction of grain into our diets on a massive scale some 10,000 years ago was another huge failed experiment.

Thyroid hormone is another example for which reference numbers of "normal" levels don't always line up with standard ranges. Many people criticize the fact that low-carbohydrate diets are associated with lower levels of circulating thyroid hormone, which often leads people to promote regularly refeeding with large carbohydrate doses to "rescue" thyroid function. Unfortunately, we have too many people who have a little bit of knowledge about lab tests for thyroid hormone, and they've established a "normal" reference range, but these people don't understand what the clinical context of the information means. Low levels of thyroid hormone can be completely normal as long as clinical function (a person's energy, mood, skin condition, and so on) is fine. Thyroid hormone, particularly T3, seems not to be needed as much when a person restricts carbohydrates. Often, people on low-carbohydrate diets may have a lower circulating T3 level, but they're still completely normal in terms of clinical function, and they don't need to take pills or ingest more carbohydrates. In other words, you don't need to take a pill for a symptom you don't have just because of the numbers on a lab test.

The Case for the Carnivore Diet as "Treatment"

The top three issues I've observed being improved by a carnivore diet are joint pain, digestive health, and mental health. The likely reason for this is because these issues are among the most common ailments. Mental health disorders are often given a special place in the landscape of human disease, probably because of the emotional turmoil associated with them. However, mental health issues are just diseases, as diabetes and arthritis are. Given that, no one should get upset when someone suggests that nutrition may play a role in the development or mitigation of these diseases, but some people do. Why is it considered radical to suggest that a diet of processed seed oil, grains, and oxalates is linked to depression? I just don't understand that reaction.

Let me offer an example of the connection between diet and mental health from my personal experience. In summer 2018, I visited my sister and my young niece. My sister had just recently gone through a divorce and was doing the best she could with the circumstances. Her daughter was, to put it diplomatically, not being the most polite kid on the planet. Anyway, I observed a lot of tension in the house, and I asked my sister if she would consider switching her diet. She was in favor of trying it. Even though she bought products that were organic and natural, they were still processed and sugary, so we got rid of all the junk food in the house. My niece, who was nine at the time, was not happy to see us throwing out all the food; and she was on the floor rolling around and screaming (which shows the addictive nature of some of these exquisitely engineered foods). I'm happy to report that since my sister changed her approach to buying and cooking food, my niece's behavior has completely turned around. Including more animal products and little to no engineered foods in their diets was an extremely powerful behavioral intervention.

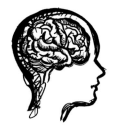

Examinations of depressed patients show that they often suffer from lower levels of carnitine than people who don't suffer from depression. You might recall from my discussion earlier in the book that humans can produce carnitine, but when we eat meat, our levels of it tend to increase. It's possible that the higher levels of carnitine are the reason so many people notice an improvement in mood after they've eaten a nice steak. Low cholesterol levels also are associated with higher rates of depression, as well as violence and suicide. Hyperinsulinemia has been associated with some mental health disorders, and in my informal studies, we have seen that eating a carnivore diet is often very effective in improving insulin status. Gut issues and inflammation are other ailments that are highly associated with mental health status. Guess what—a carnivore diet helps in those areas as well. In 1933, noted wilderness activist Robert Marshall wrote in his book *Arctic Village* that the people he lived with, who survived on caribou meat in the remote wilds of Northern Alaska, were the happiest civilization he had ever encountered. I had a patient who had spent eighteen years living off the land and surviving primarily on caribou meat in remote Alaska. There's even a movie about her experience—*The Year of the Caribou*. She was eighty-three when I knew her, and she told me that the happiest she had ever been and the best health she had experienced was during that time in Alaska.

Vegan propagandists often claim meat is inflammatory, and to support their claims about inflammation, they sometimes cite a study that used an isolated situation in which meat was not the only variable. We have to remember that human physiology is an incredibly complex system, and you can't take an isolated lab test or cell culture study and extrapolate it to the entire system. The best way to see whether meat is inflammatory to the human body is to feed it, and nothing else, to humans for a prolonged period to find out what happens via both clinical and laboratory assessment. (See Figure 7.1.) Contrary to what the vegans would like us to believe, as more and more people try out the carnivore diet, we have more evidence that meat is very much an anti-inflammatory diet.

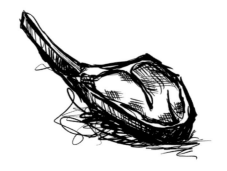

Carnivore Elimination

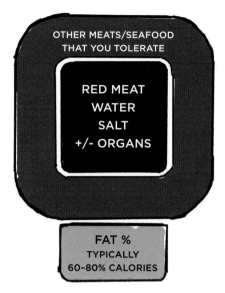

Figure 7.1
Disease mitigation

Autoimmune diseases are strongly linked with gastrointestinal problems, and increased intestinal permeability may be one of the chief culprits. Some of the recent literature on this subject focuses on altering the microbiome—often by using probiotics—to affect the intestinal permeability. This technique has generally produced little success because the microbiome is incredibly responsive to diet, and if the diet isn't altered, then the probiotic-induced shift in microbiome will likely be short-lived at best. As I previously mentioned, some of the common food components that appear to cause gut permeability issues are plant oils, drugs and supplements, legumes, grains, dairy, and sweeteners. The carnivore diet pretty much excludes all these items, except occasional limited dairy for those who can tolerate it. It's interesting to note that many people see a resolution of a variety of autoimmune conditions when they exclude those items from their diets.

Aside from the benefits that a carnivore diet has on autoimmune-related arthritis, it seems that a fairly high number of people also report improvement in the more common osteoarthritis. Conventional wisdom has been that osteoarthritis is a mechanical problem and a disease of "wear and tear." Recent studies indicate that pathophysiology of osteoarthritis has a much greater component of inflammation than previously thought, and perhaps it also has a relationship with gut permeability. A recent animal study has shown a link between carbohydrate consumption as a possible etiologic agent in osteoarthritis. So, I owe an apology to all the patients who I didn't believe when they used to tell me that eating certain foods made their joints hurt.

SUN TOLERANCE

One of the unusual side effects of a carnivore diet seems to be an increased level of sun tolerance for many, but not all, of the diet's adherents. A possible link between a decrease in consumption of omega-6 fats has been postulated as a possible mechanism. We know pre-historic man wasn't walking around with sun hats and smearing on SPF 50 sunscreen every time he went outside, so perhaps it was the meat-based diet that helped protect him from the dangers of too much sun exposure.

Common conditions such as hypertension, type 2 diabetes, and obesity often get better on a carnivore diet. These same conditions sometimes improve on other low-carbohydrate and low-calorie diets. A decrease in vascular inflammation likely contributes to improved blood pressure; often, people who have high blood pressure see improvement within a few weeks of adjusting their diets. Blood glucose stabilization typically occurs over several months. If we look at postprandial blood glucose readings of long-term carnivores, they tend to be very stable with no significant elevations, which is in contrast with what we see with most diabetics, who often have fairly wide swings in their blood glucose numbers. Likewise, overall insulin sensitivity seems to improve fairly consistently based on observation of long-term carnivore dieters who have shared their data.

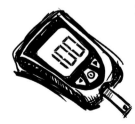

Obesity and the Carnivore Diet

Obesity is probably my least favorite subject to talk about, not because it's so contentious but because, in my opinion, it's misunderstood. Before I talk about the mechanisms by which a carnivore diet can help people to lose weight, let me explain why I think that we misunderstand obesity.

In my view, the core problem of obesity is malnutrition. We all can point to starving children who are woefully thin and agree that they're malnourished, but when we look at a morbidly obese person, malnourishment doesn't immediately spring to mind. If we look past the myriad metabolic enzymes and hormonal interactions that are constantly shifting and the issues of calorie balance and brain chemistry, we can focus on the simple fact that if the body doesn't receive proper nourishment, problems will ensue with all the bodily systems that I've talked about thus far in this chapter.

The obese are often calorie replete but nutrient starved. If you feed yourself low-quality carbohydrates that are rich in energy but low in nutrients (micronutrients, essential fats, and amino acids), you won't be satisfied. Your hunger won't be appeased, and you'll eventually fall prey to cravings for more and more food. If you continue consuming low-quality food, which is about 90 percent of what is currently available, you'll eat more and more calories and continue to suffer from what become irresistible cravings. Over time, you end up with a metabolism that doesn't work very well, a hormonal system that's suboptimal, and a severe case of carbohydrate addiction.

Many people don't believe that food is addictive, but we have ample evidence to show that certain foods stimulate the brain in ways very similar to other known addictive recreational or prescription drugs. People often mask that addiction by claiming they are "foodies" or by becoming prolific exercisers to offset the food addiction. The common platitude of "all things in moderation" is often just an excuse to get a little bit of addictive food down the gullet.

Do people lose weight because they cut calories on the carnivore diet? Yes, for some people that certainly is what occurs. Meat tends to be pretty darn satisfying and satiating to most people. Many people struggle to eat much meat, particularly when they first start the carnivore diet, and they definitely lose weight. Often, early weight loss is due to water weight coming off, particularly if a person is switching from a high-carbohydrate diet. Carbohydrates stimulate insulin to the greatest degree, which leads the kidneys to hang on to fluid that is often stored with glycogen.

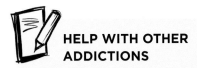

HELP WITH OTHER ADDICTIONS

Some people who've switched to a carnivore diet have found that once they've adapted and become victorious over cravings for addictive foods, they've been less inclined to indulge in other addictions, such as to alcohol and cigarettes. Many people have been able to quit using those things altogether.

Some people swear that on a carnivore diet, they eat far more than they did before, but they still lost weight. Perhaps dramatically increasing protein plays a role because protein is extremely difficult to turn into body fat, and numerous protein overfeeding studies confirm this. Is it possible that a shift in hormones due to a different food substrate plays a role either in impacting satiety or upregulating metabolic rate? Certainly, this is a hotly debated topic, and I don't pretend to know conclusively what the answer is. I know that my body handles energy expenditure in ways I have no voluntary control over. How much heat I produce is dependent upon the environment I'm in, the activity I'm engaged in, and perhaps the fuel I'm using. Many people report feeling more energized on the carnivore diet as aches and pains go away, and often they feel the desire to move a bit more often. Ultimately, I don't think the exact mechanism much matters in the grand scheme of things. When we get our bodies the correct nourishment, our health starts to thrive, and that is where the prize lies.

I come back to the topic of body composition in the next chapter where I talk about how to implement and sustain the diet, how to monitor whether it's working for you, and what kind of changes you might see when you let meat be the center of your diet.

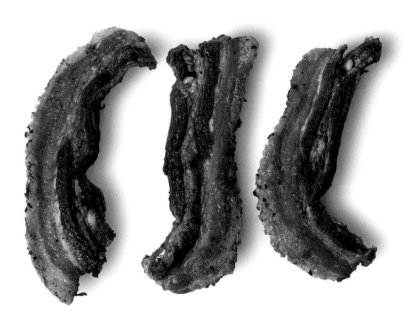

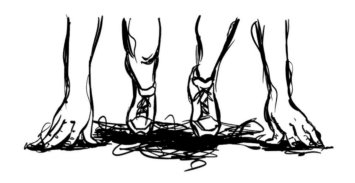

CHAPTER EIGHT

LET'S DO THIS: GETTING STARTED

Now that I've told you about the benefits of the carnivore diet and addressed some of the science behind it, I want to get into how you can implement it in your life. If I had to describe a dietary strategy to my dog, it would take about five seconds. I'd say, "Here, eat this," and that would be all he needs to thrive and be happy. Humans, on the other hand, seem like they need a lot more hand-holding. If I were to give you the kind of explanation I'd give my dog, it would go something like, "Just eat a damn steak; repeat when hungry." In fact, I could sum up this whole book with that last sentence, but I know that most people like a little more information, so I'll give you more detail.

One of the hardest concepts to understand about the carnivore diet is how simple it is. Do you need to track macros or calories? Do you need to weigh your food and calculate micronutrient amounts? Do you need to be hooked up to daily blood monitors and check your lab results every few months? I would argue that you don't need to do any of that. If a diet requires constant monitoring and calculation, then it is arguably not a very good or sustainable diet.

One big misconception about the carnivore diet is that it's a way to lose weight. Certainly, weight loss can and often does occur, but it's not guaranteed. Some folks even gain body fat. I mentioned in Chapter 7 that malnutrition is a huge problem because people tend to eat energy-rich but nutrient-poor; this diet tends to fix that imbalance. If you approach this diet with the focus of weighing a certain amount or fitting into a certain size of jeans, then you will likely struggle. It's not that those things won't happen, but they're secondary to improvements in nutrition. Nutrition precedes health; health precedes body recomposition. Sure, you can always lose weight via a variety of schemes. Cutting calories is a common approach, and it certainly can be effective in the short term and if you want to lose weight as rapidly as possible. For weight loss, there are likely better methods than a carnivore diet, particularly when a person implements it in the way I think it should be done. So if your only goal is to lose weight and you have no concern for improving aspects of your health and nutrition, you might be better served by choosing another plan.

How Should I Approach the Carnivore Diet?

Here are some simple rules for getting started:

 1. Take one day at a time. You're not committing to a life sentence when you start a carnivore diet, and you're not joining a race. Enjoy life! Each day is a new chance to learn and experiment. This experience should be about you finding out what it takes for you to feel and function your best. There is no one way to follow the plan, but there are common paths. Remember that failure precedes success, so don't beat yourself up about any miscues.

2. **Enjoy the process.** I often tell people to count how many meals they enjoy after starting the carnivore diet. You should enjoy most of your meals. If you don't enjoy what you eat, you'll never stay with any diet long term. Learning how to cook and prepare meat can be a wonderfully enjoyable process. When you're starting, variety can be your friend, so experiment with your choices. There are thousands of different cuts and types of animal products to enjoy. Find out what you like and dislike. If you love rib-eye steak and want to eat it twenty days in a row, go for it; there's nothing wrong with doing that. Are organ meats something you like? Dig in! If not, don't worry about it. If you like to season your meat, have at it. Want to add a bit of cheese on top of your burger patty? Please do. Transitioning to the diet should be an enjoyable experience.

3. **Eat enough.** The vast majority of issues that occur with transitioning are a result of not eating enough. Many people come from a background of restricting calories or macronutrients, and that habit is often hard to break. That style of eating leads to a poorly regulated appetite and a ton of anxiety. (I'm going to keep repeating this idea: If you're constantly managing your appetite, you *will not* be happy.) Why do you think humans, or any other animal, has an appetite? Is it there only to torture you, make you tougher, or give you more will power? No! It's a physiologic response to a homeostatic need. When you're hungry, you should eat! (Shocking, I know.) However, think about it in the context of any other physiologic function. When you need air, you breathe. It's as simple as that, and eating to satisfy hunger can be the same. When you're eating a species-appropriate diet, you will find that once you become healthy, your appetite will become very well regulated. (I talk more about that "once you become healthy" qualifier later in this chapter when I discuss ways you can modify the carnivore diet after you've become fully adapted to it.) While adapting to the diet, eat until you're full, and repeat as often as needed to keep yourself out of the cupcakes. If you try to limit your intake, you'll rapidly fall prey to old habits and cravings. It's a tough world out there, and temptation is everywhere; few people have the mental discipline to resist when the physiology is not favorable. Stack the deck in your favor and keep yourself constantly sated with meat. Soon your cravings will go from an irresistible gale force wind to a tiny breeze.

4. **Don't make comparisons.** Your results are *your* results, and they may be different than someone else's. Constantly comparing yourself to others is a quick path to misery. Be objective about who you are, where you're starting, and what's important to you. You're more than a number on a scale or a collection of lab values. Your physiology is dynamic and unique to your environment. Yes, we're all humans and share the same basic physiology.

Although many commonalities exist, a lot of variables go into what makes you who you are. People tend to get hung up on body image. Human beings did not evolve as fitness models or bodybuilders, and the desire to look a certain way has given us a distorted view of what may be optimal as far as health and function are concerned. If you have mostly aesthetic goals, a carnivore diet can be a tool to get where you want to be, but much, much more goes into that process than just getting healthy. Instead of focusing on the outward physical aspect, focus on the simpler goal of restoring normal health, which is something few people enjoy these days. Reflect why you're considering a dietary change and what you hope to achieve both in the short and long terms, and keep those personal goals in mind as you go on your journey.

5. You're eating for you. The pressure to fit in socially can sometimes be enormous, and many people collapse on a diet so as not to disappoint a friend or loved one. People who truly care for you will understand that you're embarking on a trial to improve some aspect of your being, and they'll respect what you're doing. You shouldn't have to defend your dietary choices, but unfortunately, sometimes it's unavoidable. If someone questions you about your bunless burger, all you have to say is, "It's what I want to eat."

6. Focus on feasting. One currently popular trend is to go long periods without eating. Time-restricted feeding windows, intermittent fasting, and extended fasting are very much in vogue. The basis for this movement is recent literature that demonstrates that a prolonged period without food starts a process called *autophagy* in which cells recycle damaged or non-functioning cellular components in the absence of recent nutrition. As I said in rule 3, you need to eat enough, and I'm referring to both the frequency and the quantity. After some time on the carnivore diet, most people tend to fall into a pattern of eating meals less frequently. I typically eat once or twice per day, but that presumes I've eaten enough not to be hungry between feedings. If you focus on the delicious food and ensure you get plenty of it, you won't need to set a stopwatch to tell you when to eat again. When you don't eat enough, your body will let you know, and you should listen. A common theme with the carnivore diet, as you may have noticed, is to let things happen. Your body knows how to take care of itself. If you're ravenous for three days in a row, don't be afraid to feed that need. Things will level out eventually. With time, you learn to have power over food and understand what nutrition means rather than being a slave to convention or food addiction.

7. Not everything is diet related. As you become more attuned to how you respond to food, particularly as your diet begins to become narrower, it's sometimes easy to fall into the trap of analyzing every single health-related issue and trying to attribute it to diet. Diet is hugely important, and I can't overstate its effect on your health. However, constantly worrying about every blemish, belch, or sneeze is not productive and will turn you into a miserable hypochondriac. Things will happen—many good, some bad. Some will be diet-related; many will not. Take the big-picture view and learn to relax. Put your energy into thinking, "How does my health compare to three months ago?" rather than thinking, "How does my health compare to yesterday?"

What Should I Eat?

I'm sure you've been thinking, "What food can I eat?" Generally, if a food comes from an animal, you can eat it: beef, lamb, chicken, turkey, deer, bison, fish, shellfish, pork, caribou, whale, shark, elephant, snake, crocodile, whatever. Most people on a carnivore diet limit what they eat to the animals that are available in the same geographic region where they live. Eggs work for many people, but they're problematic for other people. I recommend that you use eggs as a side dish, perhaps in the classic form of steak and eggs for breakfast. I eat eggs once in a while—often when I'm traveling. In general, they're a nutrient-rich food, and they make for a nice addition to your meals if you tolerate them.

Dairy is unpredictable. Some people do poorly with it, perhaps because of lactose intolerance or some other sensitivity. Other people find they can handle nonbovine dairy foods, such as sheep's or goat's milk dairy. Other people claim to do better with raw dairy or A2 dairy (dairy that contains only A2 beta-casein). Remember: Like many plant foods, dairy was relatively a late addition to the human diet. If you struggle with health issues, I strongly recommend that you consider forgoing dairy for at least a trial period.

Aside from different tolerances to the various types of dairy, people sometimes find they tolerate some dairy styles better than others. For example, many people tolerate hard cheeses better than they tolerate softer cheeses or milk. Some people don't tolerate cheese or milk, but butter and especially ghee don't cause any problems for them. Fermented dairy products, such as kefir and yogurt, can be fine for some people but cause issues for others. If you choose to use these products, don't use the varieties with added flavoring or sugars. I'm not convinced you always need to choose high-fat products versus other products; it depends on the ingredients. If the food includes a lot of gums, stabilizers, or sweeteners, I generally avoid it.

People often ask me about cooking oils. My simple answer is that you should use animal fats, period. Use butter, ghee, lard, tallow, suet, duck fat, and so on. Plant oils are generally garbage for us; there's no need for them. And, honestly, the animal fats taste and cook better anyway. My apologies to any keto folks in the audience, but I suggest you dump the coconut oil, MCT oil, avocado oil, and olive oil. Although these oils are generally better options than corn, soybean, and canola oils, they still can contain compounds that might be problematic—for example, salicylates in coconut oil, which, cause a rash, digestive upset, headaches, or swelling for some people. Here's a trick I often use when I'm cooking: Heat a pan. Touch the fatty edge of the meat I'm cooking to the pan until the fat melts. By doing this, I get a nice layer of fat to cook the meat in.

Spices and seasonings come in handy, especially for people who are transitioning into the carnivore diet. Many people do fine with spices and seasonings over the long term, although just as many people tend to find them less desirable over time. I often use only salt on my steaks, and I'm quite happy with that. Sometimes I add some spice to the meats and consider the meal to be a bit of a special occasion. I suggest you avoid sauces that are heavily laced with sugar, vegetable oils, soy, gluten, MSG, and other ingredients that have the potential for problems. If you want to add flavor to your meats, the best option is to make homemade rubs, spice blends, or marinades. Cooking with herbs or vegetables also can add a nice flavor, but you need to be objective about how they affect you and eliminate anything that causes a problem.

Carnivore Basic

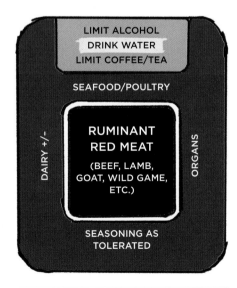

Figure 8.1
Beginning to transition
to carnivore

Red meat and water is the basis.
Fat % should be 50–80% most of the time.

What Should I Drink?

Every animal on the planet drinks water; it works well for hydration. Seventy percent of your body is made of water. It's all you need to drink, and as you get unhooked from sugar and artificial sweeteners, you'll come to enjoy it. If you want to go crazy, get some sparkling water. Although you might feel like you might die at first, you really and truly won't perish if you don't have some kind of sweet beverage to drink. Water—it's good. Drink it!

What about bone broth, alcohol, and coffee? Bone broth is fine. It contains some good stuff and can help to satisfy your urge to drink something hot or flavored. However, drinking bone broth isn't crucial to the success of the carnivore diet. You don't need to drink it unless you want to. You can get all the nutrients you need without it, but if you enjoy or benefit from it, feel free to indulge.

Alcohol is not a health food. It won't make you live longer, and it won't make you any hardier. When you're deciding whether to indulge in alcohol or skip it, understand that ethanol is toxic. Once in a while, I have a glass of red wine or two. I generally can expect my sleep to be less restful, and my athletic performance often is a little impaired the next day. Neither issue is the end of the world; the important thing is that I understand what the negative consequences of having the wine are and account for them when I make my decision. Most people who do a carnivore diet for a long period report their desire to drink alcohol drastically diminishes. Beer and certainly sugary mixed drinks are a bigger negative than a dry wine or a distilled spirit. Some people even have problems with the grains that are distilled to make the liquor.

Coffee is something I have little experience with. I've tried a few cups here and there over the decades, but I've never enjoyed it. Perhaps, if you're a coffee lover, my inexperience is reason enough for you to stop listening to me. Many people find coffee incredibly satisfying and often turn drinking it into a ritualistic experience.

The science on whether coffee is good or bad for us continually changes. Caffeine has some effects on our physiology and acts as a central nervous system stimulant. It also affects the sympathetic nervous system and has been shown to aid in sports performance. However, research has found that it leads to sleep disturbance and can negatively affect gastrointestinal motility and gastric acid secretion. Some people find that caffeine acts to dysregulate appetite, often suppressing it. It may interfere with nutrient and mineral absorption. In all likelihood, though, for most people caffeine

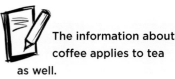

The information about coffee applies to tea as well.

probably has a minimal impact in the grand scheme of things My suggestion is that you not try to quit coffee or caffeine during the initial phases of the diet. Once you've adapted to your new eating habits, give it a go if it's something you want to take on.

How Much Should I Eat?

This question is perhaps more common than any other question I receive. My smart-aleck answer often is, "Enough." Although that might sound flippant, it's truly a very honest and simple answer. But how do you know what is enough?

I'm going to throw out some general numbers; don't take these as gospel. I'm merely giving you some ballpark starting figures; they aren't concrete figures that you have to apply:

- **Males:** Around 2 pounds of meat per day

- **Females:** Around 1.5 pounds of meat per day

When you first start, aim for the suggested amount and then adjust as needed. For instance, many small females can put away 4 to 5 pounds of meat in a day without a problem. I don't think you should shy away from that quantity if your appetite directs you there for a while. More often than not, females have a long history with diet and caloric or nutrient restriction, and they have some catching up to do to replenish their bodies with nutrients.

Remember, protein is used to build our bones, internal organs, muscles, and skin. If those tissues are depleted, plenty of food is necessary to bring them back to normal function. Also, remember that weight loss is not the short-term goal of the carnivore diet; instead, get healthy and stop with the constant anxiety created by day-to-day fluctuations in weight. Just relax and enjoy the freedom of eating. If you eat and find that you're still hungry, eat more. If you find your energy or performance is lagging, then eat more. If you find your mood is low, then eat more. The typical gnawing in the stomach and the "I've gotta eat something in the next five seconds or someone is going to get hurt" sensation of hunger will go away. Hunger often becomes a subtle signal that maybe you should eat something soon rather than it being a sign of cellular crisis of impending glucose depletion.

How Often Should I Eat?

In the beginning, your meal frequency should be whatever it needs to be to keep you satisfied. Do you feel peckish an hour after throwing down a 24-ounce porterhouse steak? Fire up another steak or line up a pound of bacon. Do what it takes to quench your appetite. Beat back the craving demons and learn to fill up on nutrition, not entertainment. Over time, you'll find that your cravings will diminish; eventually, they'll likely disappear. At that point, you'll see the emergence of a regular, well-regulated appetite that meets your nutritional needs. I know I keep saying this over and over again, but the carnivore diet isn't a quick-weight-loss scheme. Trying to fix a malnutrition problem by starving yourself is a recipe for disaster. If your goal is to lose 20 pounds, and instead you gain 5, but you now enjoy life, don't have back pain, and are no longer a slave to processed food, you're far better off with the 5 extra pounds for now.

What Does a Meal Plan Look Like?

You may be wondering what a few typical meals look like for someone who's following the carnivore diet. An average-sized rookie male carnivore who pursues an average level of activity might have a meal plan that looks like this:

Day	Meal 1	Meal 2	Snacks
1	Eggs and bacon	New York strip steak	Homemade jerky
2	Salmon	Rib-eye steak	Hard-boiled eggs
3	Hamburger patties with cheese	Chicken thighs	Pork rinds
4	T-bone steak and eggs	Lamb chops	Pemmican
5	Brisket	Liver	Cheese
6	Sardines and burger patties	Pork shoulder	Leftover steak
7	Rib-eye steak	Rib-eye steak	Bacon

The food items are pretty simple stuff, and he eats his meals as often as needed in the quantity needed to keep himself full. If he has a craving for something sweet, he could conquer it with a few pieces of already-cooked bacon or some previously cut-up steak. As I said before, it's far better to overeat in the beginning than to eat too little. I often tell people, "Eat meat like it's your job." Eventually eating meat will be more like a hobby, but in the beginning, you might have to attack it with more discipline.

How Do We Define Health?

Let's talk about health for a minute. How do we even define it? Is it something that your doctor determines by taking some blood and checking an X-ray? Or is *health* more accurately defined as the absence of disease? Think about when you were young. Hopefully, you were full of energy, life was fun, and you were free from joint pain, digestive problems, and skin problems. We expect that with age comes pain and disability. We see our peers have high blood pressure, back and knee pain, and too much body fat. Often, they are depressed and on numerous medications or supplements. These conditions become the new normal, and the situation is both expected and unquestioned.

Modern medicine has had some amazing positive benefits to society. Acute care is often outstanding, and it's saved and prolonged countless lives. Unfortunately, our record with chronic disease management has largely been an abysmal failure. Sure, we can lessen symptoms a little bit. A doctor can give you a pill to lessen your pain (until the dose wears off). If you have high blood pressure, there's a pill to lower it. If you have diabetes, no problem; we have pills and shots ready for you. Feeling depressed? Yep, there's a pill for that. Did that pill kill your sex drive? That's okay. We have other pills that take care of that. And so it goes.

I think this cycle is tragic and reflects poorly on my profession. I sometimes hear politicians debating the various ways to pay for the ever-growing health disaster. Instead of worrying about that, how about we stop making so many damn sick people! Stop feeding them garbage; you *do not* grow a healthy population on granola bars, soybean oil, and bananas. Human beings thrive on meat; it's *that* simple. If we're going to have a healthy population, we need to focus on true health rather than on managing diseases. We provide no more than lip service to the concept of prevention.

Billions of dollars in pharmaceuticals and technology are spent to put high-tech, expensive bandages on diseases. Prevention gets a pittance in spending, and no one gets reimbursed worth a darn for focusing on it.

I probably could rant on this subject enough to fill an entire book, so I should get back to defining health. Here is *my* opinion, and I think many people will agree: When I am healthy, I am free of pain, and my physiologic processes work as designed with efficiency and without issue. My energy is good, my mood is stable, and I'm generally happy and hopeful. My skin is free from itching, cracking, or rashes. My desire and capacity to exercise are good. My joints and muscle function well and are free of pain. My libido is good, as is my sexual function. My body composition is within a healthy range, and I can maintain that range without constantly being hungry. I'm sure you could add other ideas to this list as well, but I think I've made my general point.

The 100-meter sprint record for the men's 85-year-old category is about 15 seconds. If I line up fifty males spanning a range of ages and ask them to run 100 meters, the ones who can do it in less 15 seconds are far more likely to live longer than those who can't. I think this is fairly obvious to most people, but it deserves more research.

Most of the people who would "pass" this test would be younger, and that makes sense. Younger people are likely to live longer than older people because they tend to have less disease burden. But what if we had a twenty-year-old who could run it in 22 seconds and a forty-year-old who could do it in 12 seconds? What differences are there between them? To run fast, you can't be too obese, and you have to have a fairly decent body composition. Your muscles need to be strong enough to propel your body weight down the track. Joint pain or other joint problems are going to slow you down. If your cardiorespiratory fitness is compromised, you'll likely fade halfway through the run. If your flexibility is poor, you'll likely lack the range of motion necessary to reach sufficient speed. When we go into the wild and watch a prey animal getting culled by predators, the animals that typically fall victim are the slow, injured, or weak ones. Humans typically don't need to worry about being eaten by a bear, but becoming slow, weak, or otherwise physically impaired hastens our demise anyway. Instead of running from a bear, we're running from cancer, heart disease, or dementia.

What Kind of Changes Can I Expect?

Before I launch into what kind of changes might happen for your health, let me review the basic beginner rules:

 Eat meat to satiety, repeat as necessary.

 Use a variety of animal foods, including eggs and dairy as needed.

 Enjoy your meals.

 Don't undereat.

 Season meat as needed to keep it palatable.

 Put away your scale and calculator. The goal is nutrition, not some arbitrary number on the scale or a specific dress size.

Here are a couple of thoughts that I didn't state before, but they're just as important as the others:

 Don't beat yourself up if you go off plan.

 Don't stress about minute details.

Now, you're probably wondering what kind of problems you may run into as you transition, and you need to know what to do about them. Transitioning from one thing to another can be difficult. It doesn't matter where you're starting or where you're going. Changes in relationships, jobs, and family situations are challenging, and diet is the same. The transition period is a stressful time on your physiology, and problems can often manifest in several ways. A new diet, regardless of its composition, affects gut function, causes a stress response, and induces some metabolic changes. But I can give you some ideas of what to expect and how to handle any issues.

Fatigue

One of the most common issues of the transition period to a carnivore diet is fatigue, lethargy, or poor energy. As you ramp up your metabolic machinery to deal with a new fuel source, you initially will be fairly inefficient. Your capacity to extract all the nutrition from meat may be compromised. Many people suffer from decreased stomach acid production or other digestive maladies, and those issues may take a while to resolve after you transition to a carnivore diet. While your body works on resolving those issues, you may find that you can't eat as much as you need to, or perhaps you'll eat quite a bit but won't fully absorb it. Whether you're undereating or not making use of all that you do eat, a lack of adequate calories and other nutrients can lead to poor energy or fatigue. Eating more is the most helpful solution for this, and it's what I suggest as the first line of treatment. Increasing your meal frequency and adding salt to your diet often allow you to eat a bit more. For some people, digestive enzymes—like lipases, proteases, or HCl supplements—aid with the transition period. Most people can discontinue them after a few weeks.

Bowel Movements

Malabsorption, typically of fat, can often show up as steatorrhea, or fatty, loose stools. As you transition to the carnivore diet, your microbiome goes through a shift in its composition. The fiber-loving magical bacteria in your gut dies off and is replaced with meat-loving bacteria. One of the more common digestive issues as this happens is not constipation but diarrhea.

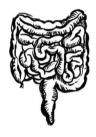

Constipation is the inability to have a complete evacuation of stool from the lower intestine. In other words, you have a bunch of fecal matter in your colon, and you can't pass it. This is the opposite of what typically happens on a carnivore diet. You might have heard the myth about meat rotting in one's colon, but what actually occurs is that meat is almost completely absorbed in the small intestine, and only a very small amount of liquid remains to enter the large intestine. Researchers have confirmed this process via studies of ileostomy patients who have had their colons removed for various disease conditions.

Most people on a high-fiber diet are accustomed to daily (and often multiple daily) bowel movements. Going on a carnivore diet will dramatically reduce the volume of waste you produce, and it will likely lead to less frequent bowel movements. Think of all the money you'll save on water and toilet paper! What many people mistake for constipation, particularly early on in the diet, is just a dramatic reduction in waste. Instead of seeing half the organic fruits and vegetables that you paid a premium price for going down the toilet as indigestible fiber, you now will produce a tiny fraction of waste. If you're habituated to going to the toilet every day or at a certain time each day, and you find that on a carnivore diet nothing comes out, you may think you're constipated. Really, though, your habit is changing because there's not much in your colon. You can still hide in the bathroom and check the latest updates on social media, but you might not produce anything while you're in there. It's not uncommon for people to go several days (and perhaps a week or more) without having a bowel movement. If you're not having discomfort or pain when you have a bowel movement, you don't have anything to be concerned about. Some people find that adding a bit more dietary fat or avoiding dairy can help things move a bit quicker. Can you suffer from true constipation while you're on the carnivore diet? Sure, but it's not common, and sometimes it's a result of an electrolyte issue that has caused altered gut motility. Adding fat, fluids, and sometimes electrolytes can be helpful.

As I mentioned earlier, for people on the carnivore diet, diarrhea is a more common issue than constipation. Several factors contribute to the issue. In addition to storing waste material, the colon has a pretty important role in absorbing fluid and electrolytes from your waste. When you're on a high-fiber diet, the relative amount of fluid entering the colon is low compared to the amount of solid material. When you're on a carnivore diet, that situation reverses. Now your colon, which has been used to dealing with a relatively small quantity of liquid leaving the small intestine, needs to adjust to receiving material that's almost completely liquid. This situation is a bit like a boxer who's been sitting on the couch for a year and suddenly has to get ready for a fight; it takes a while for him to get back into shape. Your colon has to ramp up capacity to deal with a greater amount of fluid than it's been used to. More often than not, this issue will resolve on its own if you give it time. However, if you want to minimize the possibility of experiencing the issue, things in the carnivore diet that are most likely to contribute to diarrhea are eggs, pork, and too much or too little fat. Sometimes certain spices, sauces, or marinades cause problems. Some people gradually wean off fiber over a period instead of switching into a full-on carnivore diet, and the more gradual pace allows the colon to adjust without producing diarrhea.

GERD and Gallbladder

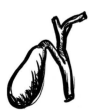

Gastroesophageal reflux disorder (GERD) is a common condition for many people. In most cases, the carnivore diet seems to clear up this problem. However, some people find that the diet makes reflux worse or that nausea or other types of dyspepsia occur.

For some people, fat, or perhaps meat in general, is difficult to digest. Strategies to deal with this problem include lowering the fat content a bit and temporarily adding digestive aids as you go through the transition period. Hydrochloric acid supplements (most commonly betaine HCl) or a bile supplement (like ox bile) can be effective. Some people notice that not drinking water around mealtimes can help; the theory is that water in the stomach dilutes the stomach acid and decreases the acidity of the stomach, which leads to difficult digestion. Some people have observed that adding salt to their diet helps with symptoms of reflux as well.

While we are on this general topic, I want to point out that many people who are without a gallbladder successfully manage quite well on a carnivore diet. The gallbladder stores bile, which acts as a detergent to emulsify fats for easier digestion in the small intestine. Without a gallbladder, the liver still produces bile, but the bile isn't released in a bolus fashion in response to a fatty meal as it would be in the presence of a functioning gallbladder. Interestingly, the common bile duct often expands chronically after gallbladder removal and can "store" a little bile for release, sort of like a mini gallbladder. Folks who have had their gallbladders removed often initially use lipases and bile supplements, limit fat, or eat smaller, more frequent meals as they transition to the carnivore diet.

OTHER DIGESTIVE SYSTEM CONCERNS

Former bariatric and gastric bypass patients are other special groups of people who may have to modify meal frequency and portion size. I know of numerous people successfully doing a carnivore diet post-bariatric surgery. In some cases, a person who's had bariatric surgery needs to supplement certain nutrients because some types of surgery result in the loss of some absorptive capacity. If you've had bariatric surgery, you may be at added risk for vitamin or mineral deficiency and need to supplement.

Patients who've had lower intestinal resections because of conditions like Crohn's disease, ulcerative colitis, or cancer often report excellent function while adopting a fully carnivore diet. People with active disease or conditions like irritable bowel syndrome can have a tumultuous transition to the carnivore diet. However, they usually note a gradual and steady overall improvement, although it can take many months for things to smooth out.

Joint Pain and Gout

For the vast majority of carnivore converts, joint pain or other musculoskeletal pain diminishes or goes away completely. A small subset of people reports a temporary increase in pain as they first start the diet. One possible reason for this phenomenon of more pain is higher uric acid levels. We know that elevated uric acid levels are associated with gout, and a diet that puts someone into ketosis can sometimes lead to increased uric acid levels. The uric acid level likely increases because the body is inefficient at using the ketones, so for a while, more ketones are excreted as waste in the urine. The ketones the kidney excretes can competitively inhibit the excretion of uric acid, so the level of uric acid rises and potentially results in joint pain or other pains.

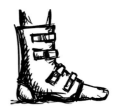

Over time, your body becomes more efficient at using the ketones you produce, and you tend not to waste as much through the urine. The uric acid levels often normalize, and the joint pain disappears. In fact, the vast majority of gout sufferers who do a carnivore diet long term find their gout symptoms vanish. Remember, the Inuit, Maasai, and other meat-dependent tribes weren't known for having problems with gout. Historically, people with gout have been wealthy and have indulged in sugar, alcohol, and meat. Eliminating sugar and alcohol from the diet seems to go a long way toward eliminating gout. If you're predisposed to gout attacks, one strategy you can use during a transition period is to prophylactically take medication for treating gout during the transition period.

People often report a change in their breath. This is because acetone can be wasted via the breath when it's present at relatively high levels, and the smell can be noticeable. This issue tends to go away as the body better adapts to using ketones.

Skin Conditions

Some people report that they develop a rash as they transition to the carnivore diet, but the incidence seems fairly rare. Skin issues are likely related to the elimination of ketones (as I describe in the previous section). In this case, the body excretes the ketones through the skin, which results in an irritation response. Skin conditions usually resolve with time as the body becomes more efficient with using ketones.

Headaches

One transition-phase issue I dealt with was headaches. Headaches are most likely related to fluid and electrolyte shifts that occur as your body adjusts to the new eating regimen. In my case, the headaches were sporadic and very mild; I had them off and on for about ten days. For those who experience headaches when they first start the carnivore diet, I recommend eating more food and upping fluid and electrolyte intake. Even if you don't alter your habits, the headaches generally pass fairly quickly.

Muscle Cramps

Muscle cramps are another fairly common occurrence that seems to crop up with some regularity among carnivore dieters. Electrolyte or hydration problems may be at play here. For most people, the cramps dissipate with more time on the diet. I've been following the diet for almost two years, and I get an occasional muscle cramp, but I can almost always relate it to having exercised very hard and without eating at an appropriate time in relation to my exercise. Eating relatively soon after you exercise—at least within a few hours—can sometimes help reduce the occurrence of muscle cramps.

Some people find electrolyte supplementation helpful, but others see little benefit in it. People have tried adding regular salt (sodium chloride), potassium, and magnesium and have found varying results. Some people soak in Epsom salts to alleviate muscle cramps.

If you experience cramps, the first thing I suggest you do is to look at your overall food intake to ensure it's adequate. Beyond that, you can add various electrolytes in the form of salt (such as Redmond Real Salt) or electrolyte supplement. Some people who exercise find that supplementing with electrolytes before working out is an effective strategy. Interestingly, many long-term carnivore dieters go without any added salt at all in their diets, and they seemingly do very well. Because salt can act as an appetite stimulant and lead to excessive eating, I recommend you use salt as needed, using taste as a guide.

Ketosis

If you've done any research on the ketogenic or other low-carbohydrate diets, you've probably heard of ketosis, so let me talk a bit about it and how it relates to the carnivore diet.

The point of the carnivore diet is not to achieve a state of constant ketosis, and artificially manipulating fat ratios is not part of the program. Many people, if not most, who measure their blood ketones notice a moderate amount of ketones being produced, and the amount is often more than the theoretical threshold of "nutritional ketosis," which is 0.5 millimoles per deciliter of blood. I believe it's counterproductive to measure ketones because it usually leads to unnecessary anxiety and a waste of money that you could otherwise spend on food.

If you have a medical condition that requires you maintain a minimal level of ketones, you're in a different situation. For most folks, though, I recommend putting away both the ketone monitor and the scale. Measuring ketones, especially if you're coming from a ketogenic diet background, can push you away from eating enough protein, or it leads you to gorge on unnecessary added fats, and neither of those situations is desirable. Our ancestors thrived on a carnivore diet without worrying about ketone levels, and you can, too. Remember, your ultimate goal is to be in a position where appetite and eating are naturally controlled, and you're not constrained by some arbitrary number or a predetermined fasting window.

Energy Level

Many people say they notice a general increase in their energy and work or exercise capacity. This rise in energy level often comes even as sleep quantity decreases. People often state that they have very restorative sleep, but the overall quantity of sleep they get decreases. They may wake up

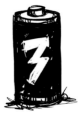

before the alarm goes off but feel rested and ready to go. My sleep volume reduced by about 15 percent, but I didn't experience any loss of energy or performance. Perhaps people on the carnivore diet require less sleep because they have better materials with which to repair their bodies, and they might be less beat up metabolically.

However, not everyone immediately has deep, restorative sleep as soon as they transition to the carnivore diet. Some people have a hard time sleeping, particularly early on. Some people feel the need to urinate, and it wakes them up at night. Eating more protein can require more water for processing the food, which can lead to increased thirst. Drinking more to satisfy the thirst leads to increased urination. Salt ingestion also likely plays a role here. One strategy that can help is moving the last meal of the day to an earlier time (if that plan is practical for your schedule and allowed by your appetite). A fair amount of emerging circadian biology research indicates that eating the bulk of our food during the daylight hours may be beneficial. Modulating salt intake might be another strategy for preventing fluid shifts at night.

Other people have a feeling of too much energy that keeps them wired and awake. It's important to employ standard sleep hygiene practices. Here are some guidelines:

 Don't exercise within a few hours of planned sleep.

 Shut off electronics an hour or so before going to bed. Artificial light, particularly blue light, is thought to lead to sleep disturbances.

 Sleep in a cool environment.

 Don't drink alcohol.

COOLING DOWN

I often take a cool shower within an hour of going to bed because it can help to bring down my core body temperature. A lower core body temperature is one of the signals our bodies use to indicate we're ready for sleep.

How Do I Transition to the Diet?

Now I'm ready to give you some more detail about common strategies to transition into the diet. There are pros and cons to these methods, and no solution is going to fit everyone. Your starting diet may help dictate which method you want to pursue.

Hard-Core Carnivore

This method is pretty much a direct drop into the purest form of the diet. If you go hard-core carnivore, you go straight to meat and water all the time right from the get-go. Many long-term carnivores recommend using this technique, which is analogous to removing a bandage by quickly ripping it off. There might be more discomfort in the short term, but the overall process often is quicker than easing into the diet.

With this method, on day one, you start eating nothing but meat and drinking nothing but water, and you repeat until you've adapted. This approach works best for very motivated individuals and those who are transitioning from a mostly animal-based ketogenic diet (because they're already pretty well accustomed to fueling on fat).

The downside of this cold turkey approach for many people is that the symptoms associated with the transition can be more severe than with a more gradual switch. Consequently, some people quit because the transition is too difficult.

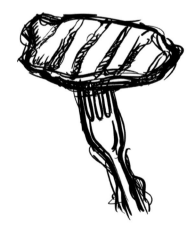

Carb Step-Down Strategies

If you're coming from a carbohydrate-heavy background, a good strategy may be to first adopt a lower-carbohydrate diet for at least several weeks before transitioning to a full carnivore diet.

If you've been on a standard American diet, which is high in carbohydrates, and you've been taking medications to address high blood pressure, diabetes, chronic pain, or depression, you should visit with your physician to discuss potential medication changes that might need to occur as you shift your diet. I'll use blood pressure medication as an example: Many people find that medications to treat blood pressure can lead to dangerously low blood pressure as your body adapts because the diet can normalize blood pressure. The result is that the medication becomes unnecessary or needs to be reduced. The body can make similar adjustments for the other types of ailments, and it's important that you and your doctor make corrections to your medication as necessary.

Six-Week Carnivore Transition

WEEK 1	3 FULL-CARNIVORE MEALS
WEEK 2	8 FULL-CARNIVORE MEALS REDUCE DIETARY FIBER BY 25%
WEEK 3	10 FULL-CARNIVORE MEALS INCLUDING 2 FULL-CARNIVORE DAYS
WEEK 4	5 FULL-CARNIVORE DAYS REDUCE DIETARY FIBER BY 50%
WEEK 5	85% FULL-CARNIVORE WEEK ALL BUT 2 FULL-CARNIVORE MEALS REDUCE DIETARY FIBER BY 75%
WEEK 6	100% CARNIVORE WEEK NO MORE DIETARY FIBER

For some people, a good transition strategy is to include more meat-based meals gradually over time. One example schedule is to spread three fully meat-based meals throughout the first week. The next week bump up to eight carnivore meals. In the third week, try two days of only meat-based meals, and spread ten carnivore meals on the other days. In the fourth week, you should be able to handle five days of carnivore meals, and by the fifth week, all but two of your meals will be meat. In week six, your transition to full carnivore will be complete. Alternatively, you could set short-term challenges to go full carnivore three days out of a week. The next challenge is to go one full week of eating only meat. The third challenge is to go for two weeks; finally, you attempt to go carnivore for thirty days in a row. This method is pretty much what I used, and it was a fairly smooth process.

The third technique for a gradual transition is to fade the vegetables and starch off your plate as you increase the amount of meat you eat each day.

A drawback to these gradual techniques is that for some time, you still have access to addictive or otherwise problematic food, which may make it harder for you to let go of those things. It's kind of like having an alcoholic quit drinking by only having alcohol twice a week. However, as long as you continue moving closer to a fully carnivore diet, you will likely feel better, and those cravings will subside over time. Also, the gradual withdrawal of fiber- or oxalate-rich foods might make the transition easier. By gradually reducing fiber from your diet, your colon may better adapt to being able to absorb fluid and minerals efficiently. Gradually tapering from oxalate-rich foods may help you avoid a potential rapid precipitation of oxalate crystals into your joints, skin, or other tissues.

THE BEGINNER PHASE

How long does the beginner phase last? It can vary, but here are some signs that identify you as an experienced carnivore rather than a beginner:

- Food no longer rules you, and you no longer see food as a form of entertainment. Instead, it's a deeply satisfying form of nutrition.
- You have no problem passing up a food that was previously one of your favorites.
- You can go out socially and not cave to pressure to eat something just to satisfy someone else.
- Nothing other than meat seems like food.

For some people, these signs are evident within a few months. Other people need years to reach all these milestones.

Can I Modify the Diet?

There are many ways to tinker with any diet. Purist advocates of any diet discourage deviating from the plan, but some people will always make adjustments.

Many people can go for years (maybe even decades or a lifetime) eating to satiety and living on primarily fatty cuts of meat while being as happy and healthy as can be. Some people may stray from the carnivore diet only to discover that they need to stay in line with the diet to prevent a relapse into bad habits or to prevent devastating health issues from returning. It's likely that most people who try this diet will not remain purely carnivorous. Many will drift back and forth between the carnivore diet and a more standard diet; they might even hover around carnivory or near carnivory for much of their lives because they realize they get the best health and performance benefits the closer they are to being purely carnivorous, but they won't be 100 percent carnivores 100 percent of the time.

Unlike proponents of veganism, who often have ethical reasons for pursuing an all-plant diet, people who follow the carnivore diet do it for health and performance reasons. People on this diet aren't trying to save broccoli from extinction or believe that they're making the world a better place. It's not a religion or a cult; it's merely a way to try to be healthier and get optimal nutrition. Many people use the carnivore diet to solve health issues and fix problems—particularly with their gut function—so that they may gradually return other foods to their diets with no ill effect. Other people use a strict carnivore diet as an occasional tool, and some others may find they feel optimal if they're "mostly carnivore."

I generally don't recommend that you tinker with the carnivore diet until you've conquered all the demons that would keep you in beginner phase. I suggest everyone spend at least a few months being fully carnivorous before playing around with other stuff. When you're ready to start playing with the diet a little, you can use the common tinkering strategies in the following sections.

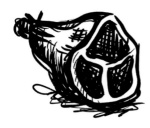

Intermittent Fasting

Intermittent fasting is an attempt to hack your appetite, and it can have benefits with the carnivore diet, but it also can result in problems. Because many people come to the carnivore diet from a background of caloric restriction, intentionally denying the body food can lead some people back into unhealthy behaviors due to excessive hunger, and I think people do better when we're not constantly snacking. Many people like eating one meal per day, which is something you can certainly do on a carnivore diet. In fact, a carnivore diet might be the diet that most lends itself to this strategy. My caveat is that you should be able to feast adequately to support your body as you go the next 24 hours without food. For some people, this may mean eating two, three, or more pounds of meat in one sitting when they have only one meal each day.

If weight loss is your goal, or you're trying to get lean beyond a normal level of body fat (which is 10 to 15 percent for men and 18 to 24 percent for women), then intermittent fasting may be helpful.

I find going much beyond 24 hours without eating to be counterproductive over the long term with this particular diet. When we're eating suboptimal or potentially toxic foods, it's often helpful to give our bodies a break. But the carnivore diet doesn't include those types of food. So if you're no longer consuming potentially harmful foods, then the benefits of extended fasting are likely diminished except in unusual cases.

I've not seen any data from studies of carnivorous animals that show benefit from fasting or caloric restriction. Specifically, athletes are unlikely to benefit from prolonged fasting, especially during competition periods. I suggest you be cautious about combining intermittent fasting with the carnivore diet.

Circadian Biology

Circadian biology deals with some of the variations that affect our physiology depending on the time of day when they occur. Night-shift workers are often observed to have poorer health markers and long-term health than people who work during the day. There is a growing body of evidence that indicates that eating during daylight hours may be preferable to eating at night. Also, many people report better sleep when their last meal of the day is not close to bedtime, and better sleep results in several other positive changes.

If you have some control over when you eat, a shift to daytime eating may yield a moderate benefit. The reality is that you should eat when you're hungry, and your work schedule often dictates when you can have your meals. If it's possible, it might be beneficial to shift your eating times. Your body most likely will acclimate to your new schedule, and your hunger will begin to coincide with the eating times you've selected.

Macronutrient Cycling

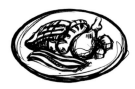

Some people have success in altering their body composition by cycling the macronutrients of fat and protein. They alternate days of eating more protein with days when they eat more fat. For example, a person could increase protein by 20 percent for three to four days and then increase fat for a day or two.

You can do this type of macronutrient cycling in the carnivore diet by eating leaner cuts of meat and then cycling in the fattier cuts. Remember that when you consciously work to alter body fat percentage to below normal levels, things become less intuitive. However, if you make slow, subtle shifts, your body usually can tolerate it fairly well.

Calories and Metabolism

Do calories matter? Yes, they do. If you burn more calories than you ingest, then you lose mass. So how do you control how many calories you burn? Also, what impacts your appetite and how many calories you take in?

This topic is the subject of much debate, with vehement advocates on both sides of the issue. Can you consciously limit your caloric intake and increase your activity level? Absolutely, and it can be an effective short-term strategy. We see the evidence all the time in the fitness community. Are there foods that are inherently more satiating than others? Again, the answer is yes, and the food industry is very aware of this fact, as evidenced by the ever-increasing number of highly palatable but ultimately unsatisfying foods that are being produced and heavily marketed. Can different people eat an identical number of calories and gain or lose different amounts of weight? Yes, of course, and one person can even see differences from one time to another. For example, compare a younger version of yourself to the current version. Which one could eat more calories without gaining weight? Most likely, it was your younger version.

Carnivore Body Composition
(not recommended until well adapted to diet)

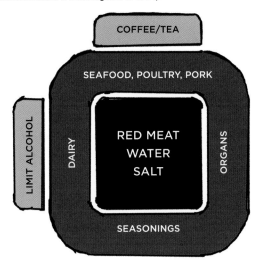

**Cycle high protein/lower fat days with higher fat days
and consider a fasting schedule**

*Figure 8.2
Body composition*

Do we have the capacity to shift our metabolic efficiency? I believe the answer is that we do, and I also believe a carnivore diet encourages some of that capacity. The benefits of the carnivore diet on metabolism are likely due to improvements in insulin sensitivity, improvements in other hormones, and cellular and mitochondrial improvements. If a person who switches to the carnivore diet can eat more food and maintain a healthy weight, similar to what that person could do while young, then he or she is likely metabolically normal. A recent $12 million one-year-long Harvard study demonstrated that people could eat around 250 extra calories per day on a low-carbohydrate diet compared to a higher carbohydrate diet and not regain previously lost weight. Additionally, numerous studies demonstrate that as protein consumption goes up, so does metabolic rate.

I often see people who follow the carnivore diet stating they're eating many more calories in meat than they ate in total before, but they're still losing weight. I don't doubt that this can occur; it likely has to do with improvements in some of the body's inefficiencies. Also, protein is particularly difficult to turn into fat metabolically. Mitochondrial density can be improved via diet, exercise, infrequent feeding, and other methods. Having more mitochondria generally means better efficiency and metabolic health. If you are hell-bent on getting to a very low level of body fat, then a combination of cycling macronutrients and a slight caloric decrease or an increase in activity can be helpful.

A strong appetite is a good sign of health, particularly when it doesn't lead to gains in body fat. Once a person hits this level of metabolic normalcy, then I believe we see more alignment with what we see in the athletic and fitness community, with a more predictable response to macronutrient compositions and caloric intake.

Carnivore Adjacent/Athletes

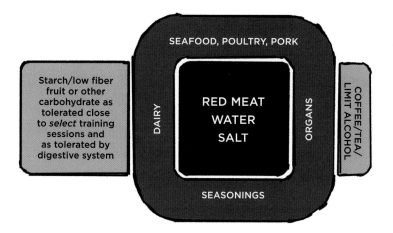

Figure 8.3
Carnivore-adjacent
athletic performance

Sporadic Use of the Carnivore Diet

For some people—particularly those who don't have significant difficulties with food addictions, cravings, or major health issues—cyclically following the carnivore diet might be a great option. This diet works well as an elimination diet. People who have problems with food sensitivity or gut health and switch to the carnivore diet likely will have eliminated the problem food. When those sensitivities have resolved after a person has been on a carnivore diet for some time, the person often can start eating other foods without ill effects. If you're in this category of people, that's great; the carnivore police aren't going to hunt you down and tell you to walk away from the blueberry or the piece of dark chocolate. However, you need to be honest with yourself. Keep in mind that none of the other foods are required for a healthy life. Meat is the basis of your nutrition. If you choose to add another type of food to your diet, you should be very objective about its effect.

Food Reintroduction

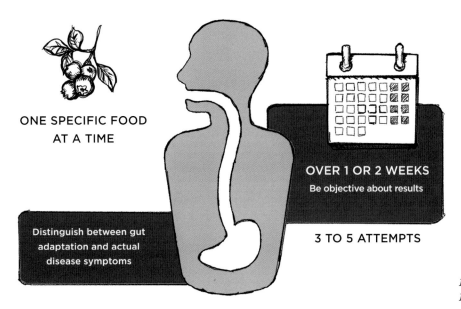

ONE SPECIFIC FOOD
AT A TIME

OVER 1 OR 2 WEEKS
Be objective about results

Distinguish between gut
adaptation and actual
disease symptoms

3 TO 5 ATTEMPTS

Figure 8.4
Food reintroduction

I recommend that you stick to single-ingredient foods as you're reintroducing items to your diet. Try eating one thing and then wait several days to assess the effect of that food. It very well may take three or more trials to get a good sense of what happens. Some adverse GI effects may simply reflect a poorly prepared gastrointestinal microbiome.

For example, let's say you've been a strict carnivore for six months, and you've taken care of all your health issues. At this point, you'd like to try occasionally having some berries. I suggest you eat a small amount one day; objectively write down any negative or positive outcomes from that trial. Wait three or four days and then repeat the process. Compare the results of the two attempts. If you seem to tolerate the berries, you can play with the quantity. You may find that a small quantity is fine, but a larger quantity is problematic.

In most cases, people who have been strict carnivores for an extended period become pretty good at assessing dietary effects on their health, mood, skin, joint pain, digestion, and so forth. After several weeks or months of trials with different foods, you should have a list of desirable and health-promoting (or at least health-neutral) foods that you can use as part of your diet on a regular or cyclic basis. If six months go by, and you find yourself a little worse for wear, you can reestablish a baseline by going back to being a strict carnivore. Surprisingly, most people who deviate from a strict carnivore diet tend to stay fairly close to the plan because they understand how powerful and satisfying the nutrition is. In other words, it's highly unlikely that a strict carnivore will eventually end up as a vegan, even though the opposite is often true.

Should I Monitor Health Markers?

Often when people follow some form of a low-carb diet, they focus on monitoring certain things through blood testing to get some insight into the effects of diet. Blood testing provides some data and often can help to troubleshoot problematic health issues. Before I get into some of the common observations that I've made about carnivore dieters, let me put some things into perspective.

When you have your blood drawn, its contents are representative of what is being transported via your blood during that exact moment in time. Many, if not most, of the things that can be measured in the blood can change on a weekly, daily, hourly, and even momentary basis. For instance, blood cholesterol can change dramatically over a few days, hormones can change by the hour, and liver enzymes or inflammatory markers can go up or down based on recent activity or exercise levels. Lab values can be significantly affected by many things, including stress, sleep, illness, activity, exercise, weather, temperature, time of day, and time of year. So, trying to attribute any one particular laboratory reading exclusively to diet can be problematic. Remember that humans are complex systems, and if you focus on an isolated variable from a single or even a few lab studies, you often miss the forest for the trees. I'm not saying you should ignore any particular lab value; instead, you should look at them in the context of the whole system.

For example, let's say my glucose is in a normal range. That may be a good thing, but it may mean I'm producing too much insulin to keep it normal. How would I know or what would lead me to suspect that it was elevated? What system-based clues might give me a hint to look further? I also need to consider whether my blood pressure is a little high, whether I have too much belly hanging over the top of my jeans, or whether my mood sucks.

Just as the nutrition science–based food recommended daily allowances were based on a population that was arguably sick from eating a high-carbohydrate, grain-based diet, many of the common laboratory reference ranges were based on that same population. We truly do not have a good set of reference ranges for the populations who follow the low-carbohydrate and carnivore diets. With this in mind, I want to share some of the areas where labs for carnivore dieters can diverge from the general population.

Blood Lipids

Blood lipids probably cause the most concern for both patients and their physicians. First of all, blood lipid levels are dynamic; they can vary fairly significantly over a matter of even a few days. Your total cholesterol on Wednesday may be remarkably different the following Tuesday. Let's assume that the numbers you get represent a daily average. (However, this assumption is likely false.) When we look at the lipid number for a carnivore dieter, we often see elevated total and LDL cholesterol; this is not always the case, and often LDL/total cholesterol will be largely unchanged or even lower. After I'd been following the carnivore diet for one year, my LDL and total cholesterol labs were largely not much different than they had been several years before when I was on a much higher carbohydrate diet. My total cholesterol was approximately 200, and my LDL was around 140.

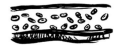

Especially during a period of weight loss, blood lipid numbers can vary because they're part of an overall energy balance and delivery system. In other words, your blood lipids can reflect the acute energy needs of your peripheral tissues. If your system is well-stocked for energy (you're in a fed state), your liver is less compelled to send out more energy via blood lipids. Seeing a high cholesterol level can be disconcerting because we've traditionally thought high cholesterol is a risk factor for cardiovascular disease in the general population. This theory was based on large population surveys, and the question we don't have the answer to is whether it applies equally to all populations, particularly people who are otherwise objectively very healthy.

Another common finding among carnivore dieters is a general trend toward elevated HDL, the so-called good cholesterol, and generally lower triglycerides. In general, higher HDL and lower triglycerides are thought to represent an improvement in cardiovascular risk, but this is not absolute, particularly regarding the HDL. As I've already mentioned, it's important that you realize that large energy shifts and weight loss can be responsible for unexpected numbers, such as higher than expected triglycerides, particularly at the beginning of a transition to the carnivore diet. I often suggest that people wait six months or more before getting routine labs after starting the diet, unless there's a compelling reason to do it earlier, such as to address an illness.

You can have more advanced lipid screening to obtain more information regarding lipid particle counts, sizes, and specialized particles. However, you have to remember that these things are dynamic and often in flux, and researchers are debating their significance.

Measuring ratios of traditional lipid panels can be used to stratify risk, and most people now concede that these ratios tend to be more helpful in identifying risk, at least in the general population, than merely looking at a single LDL or total cholesterol reading. If we think about the body as a system, then we can start to get a better handle on how things are going. Another marker that some like to use and believe is reflective of the lipid system is something called the *remnant cholesterol*, which is calculated by determining total cholesterol and subtracting both HDL and LDL to yield the remnant. Generally, the lower the remnant cholesterol number, the better. Triglyceride/HDL ratios are also a marker to take into consideration, and many find this to be a better marker of cardiovascular risk than a single LDL reading.

Glucose

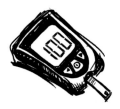

Glucose control is important, and generally speaking, a carnivore diet tends to lead to very well-controlled glucose numbers. If you're going to talk about glucose, then you definitely need to be aware of your insulin status. When you look at a blood glucose reading in isolation, you leave out a major part of the story of blood sugar control, potential diabetes, and other chronic disease risks. If you're going to worry about heart disease, insulin sensitivity is one of the most important modifiable risk factors you can be concerned with. It's right up there with smoking, and it's far more important than relative cholesterol levels. You can use a fasting insulin level with a fasting glucose level to calculate something called a HOMA-IR score, which is one of several reasonable measures of insulin sensitivity. Once again, the lower this number is, the better. Just be aware that like all labs, both glucose and insulin can vary on a daily or hourly basis.

Other ways to calculate insulin sensitivity include a triglyceride/glucose index and an LPIR score using a combination of advanced lipoprotein-testing calculations. A reasonable proxy measure for insulin sensitivity is a simple waist-to-height measurement ratio.

In general, a carnivore diet tends to lead to improved insulin sensitivity over the long term, no matter which of these methods you use to evaluate it. Glucose tends to remain stable for people on the carnivore diet because the glucose the body is using is not being ingested; it's being produced mostly from protein, a small amount of fat, and a few other sources, such as lactate, via a process generally described as gluconeogenesis. One of the more common misconceptions regarding gluconeogenesis is that it is substrate driven—that is to say, if a great deal of protein is around, then a great deal of glucose will be made. In practice, that tends not to happen, and what we see is that gluconeogenesis is primarily a demand-driven process, so glucose supply tightly matches demand. Gluconeogenesis is probably the most precise way to control glucose regulation, and in the long term, it leads to well-controlled and stable blood glucose numbers. People with both type 1 and type 2 diabetes also note that in the long term they tend to see excellent blood glucose control, although it may take a few months for the level to normalize.

One thing I want to point out is that some people will see over time that their average glucose concentration drifts up slightly, but it remains stable at that higher level. This is another reason to look at the relationship with insulin in this circumstance because it's becoming clearer that insulin may be driving diabetic pathophysiology more than it drives blood glucose. In fact, it's possible to have "normal" blood glucose numbers, but because of high levels of insulin we can start to see the occurrence of diabetic tissue damage.

Liver Function

Liver function studies tend to be normal for people on the carnivore diet, and the assumption that increased protein is damaging to the liver is based upon a fallacy. NAFLD (non-alcoholic fatty liver disease) is an increasingly common diagnosis. Fortunately, we know from observations of carnivore populations and by extrapolating data from low-carbohydrate studies that a carnivore diet tends to improve this problem. Liver function tests can be slightly elevated for several reasons, and if you're having them evaluated, you should be aware of benign reasons for their elevation. One of the more common reasons is recent intense exercise, which can result in slight elevations of these enzymes for up to a week.

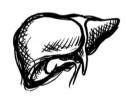

Inflammation

In a similar vein, markers of inflammation, such as C-reactive protein, can show a transient elevation after exercise or other acute stresses on the body. This marker and other inflammation labs can be used as risk factors for predicting cardiovascular or other disease potentials. Once again, it appears that a carnivore diet tends to lead to low levels of inflammatory markers.

Kidney Function

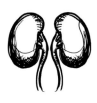

Kidney function is often a concern with higher protein diets, but the concern stems from data from animal studies that haven't been replicated with humans. In general, the consensus is that high-protein diets do not damage kidneys. Some people still are concerned that an already damaged kidney will fail more quickly in the presence of higher levels of protein, but that data is tenuous at best. We have some reports of improved renal function in people who've followed a carnivore diet. If you have compromised renal function and are concerned that consuming too much protein while on a carnivore diet might be problematic, it's worth your effort to track the function over time.

As part of the discussion about kidney function, I want to discuss a couple of labs that we might expect to be elevated but likely do not indicate a problem. Blood urea nitrogen (BUN) is often elevated on a higher protein diet, but that doesn't mean there's any problem with kidney function. This result is most likely a normal consequence of elevated protein in the diet. If there is some other reason for concern, such as pain or declining GFR (glomerular filtration rate), then you can do more formal testing. The same applies to the serum creatinine level, which also may be slightly elevated for similar reasons.

Hormone Levels

Thyroid function is generally improved on a carnivore diet, and we have observed improvements in autoimmune-related issues such as Hashimoto's thyroiditis. One interesting thing to note is that thyroid hormone, particularly T3 levels, may seem to be low, but the clinical function is noted to be good. This likely represents a decreased requirement for circulation of the hormone or an increase in receptor sensitivity. Therefore, you should not need a supplement in the absence of a clinical need.

Similarly, when people follow a carnivore diet, reproductive hormones tend to normalize and function optimally. It becomes very important to consider clinical function as we assess particular hormone levels. Most women report improved menstrual cycle regularity and resolution of things like amenorrhea or dysmenorrhea (painful periods or absence of periods). Additionally, many women have seen the resolution of polycystic ovarian syndrome (PCOS) and restoration of fertility.

Both men and women note improvements in libido and clinical testosterone function when they follow a carnivore diet, particularly after they've moved beyond the adaptation phase. Many men have reported an increase in serum testosterone levels, although this isn't always the case. Generally, however, clinical testosterone function tends to improve, and there are associated improvements in mood, sexual function, morning erections, exercise capacity, recovery from exercise, and body composition.

Iron Levels

Another theoretical concern that seems not to bear out in real-world practice are concerns about iron overload. Iron deficiency is one of the most common deficiency problems in the world, and a carnivore diet is undoubtedly the most efficacious way to prevent that problem because it's tremendously high in bioavailable heme iron. On the other hand, too much iron, particularly when stored in excess quantities in the tissue, has been associated with some health problems, such as diabetes, cardiac disease, or liver disease.

Fortunately, excess iron levels don't seem to occur to any significant degree on a carnivore diet. It's likely that underlying metabolic disease and inflammatory states contribute to excess iron storage. In general, a carnivore diet tends to improve those conditions, and that may be the reason why high storage levels as assessed by serum ferritin don't seem to be a problem, even though carnivore dieters have a relatively high iron intake.

One exception involves people who are affected by hereditary hemochromatosis, which can lead to problems with iron storage. To this point, I have not seen anyone with that condition who has had problems with the diet. However, if you suffer from hereditary hemochromatosis, it's worth closely monitoring. Making blood donations can be a strategy to offset the issue if the overall benefit of the diet is positive for you.

Miscellaneous Health Markers

In general, you can expect both red and white blood cell counts to fall within the normal ranges. However, you may see slightly lower white blood cell counts, which may be associated with a generally lower inflammatory state.

Levels of serum electrolytes, such as sodium, potassium, chloride, calcium, and magnesium, tend to be normal. Our bodies do a pretty good job of maintaining these in fairly narrow physiologic ranges.

Some people express concern that a carnivore diet can lead to an acidic environment, but our blood pH is aggressively controlled and very tightly regulated. As long as we have functioning lungs and kidneys, we can keep our blood pH right where it needs to be regardless of dietary input. The concerns about acids leaching minerals from our bones for buffering purposes are unfounded. Higher protein diets ultimately lead to better long-term bone health, especially because our bones are approximately 40 percent protein.

While I'm on the topic of unfounded concerns, the belief that a particular blood type lends itself better to meat consumption is without merit. I've surveyed hundreds of carnivore dieters, and the ones who do it successfully don't have one specific blood type in common. Largely, the frequency of successful carnivore dieters' blood types occurs with the same relative frequency as they occur in the general population. Basically, if your blood type is red, you can successfully thrive on meat. Eating meat is a conserved capacity that is shared by all humans and likely goes back many millions of years.

A couple of other genetic situations that potentially cause people to be concerned about the suitability of the diet are issues of APOE4 gene status, which has been associated with the incidence of Alzheimer's dementia, and MTHFR gene status, which interferes with a person's ability to convert homocysteine into methionine. Both of these conditions are not that uncommon, so it's unlikely that eating meat in the setting of normal metabolic health will lead to a long-term negative outcome in these situations. Monitoring things like homocysteine levels in the case of MTHFR and insulin sensitivity based on the APOE4 status are probably reasonable strategies.

Who Is the Diet Safe For?

Can a woman have a normal pregnancy on a fully carnivore diet? The short answer is yes. There are countless examples of women who have done that in modern times, and of course, we know that for thousands of years, women were doing it. It certainly makes sense to let your obstetrician be aware of your diet so you can add any recommended supplementation or other foods that you need during your pregnancy. After the baby is born, breastfeeding generally seems to go well, and problems with lactation don't seem to be common. If you're in the middle of a pregnancy, an abrupt dietary change might be stressful. I recommend you make a gradual change if you're planning on going down the path to the carnivore diet.

Children also can follow the carnivore diet. Certainly, they would have historically followed this eating style. Children don't have any different nutrition requirements than adults. In other words, kids require the same essential things that we do.

Children can begin the carnivore diet as soon as they are ready to wean off breast milk. They can begin by teething on bones and eating finely cut or pureed meats. Of course, you have to be vigilant and use caution to ensure no choking occurs.

It's often difficult to control the diet of children as they interact with their peers, and honestly kids should have a choice about what they eat; eventually, they'll be making their own decisions anyway. It helps to educate them very early on about the benefits and potential problems with food choices. At times, my children choose to be fully carnivorous, and I certainly do not discourage this practice. I ensure that they always have access to plenty of well-prepared meat dishes, which they prioritize over other foods. If they want to eat something else, such as fruit, vegetables, or other similar whole foods, after they've eaten their meat, I do not discourage them. I do limit or try to avoid exposing them to processed, sugary food, vegetable oils, and refined grain products. When they go to birthday parties or other "junk food" events, I typically send them off with full stomachs to minimize the temptation to eat a bunch of garbage. Other families have children that remain fully carnivorous, and the kids appear to be doing great.

How do athletes perform on a carnivore diet? Again, the answer appears to be that they flourish. For example, world-class athlete Owen Franks, who played for New Zealand's All Blacks rugby team, has adopted a carnivore diet. He's seen his level of performance improve and has noted greater levels of strength and lean body mass. My athletic performance has improved fairly significantly, and I've been able to set three indoor rowing masters world records and six American records since I've been fully carnivorous.

Numerous high-level athletes, including Olympic athletes, have contacted me from a variety of sports, including weightlifting, powerlifting, mixed martial arts, jiu-jitsu, CrossFit, cycling, marathon running, baseball, rowing, shot put, and rugby. All the athletes who've transitioned to the carnivore diet report significant improvement in overall performance, improved recovery, and quick healing from injury. That said, during the transition period, some athletes notice a drop in performance, which often is related to undereating or because of a need to adjust to the diet. This phase can last for several weeks to several months; the duration depends somewhat on the sport and the athlete's prior dietary strategy. For example, a person coming from a high-carbohydrate diet who engages in a highly glycolytically demanding sport such as CrossFit or cycling may take longer to adapt than other athletes. A person who was previously on a ketogenic diet and competes in powerlifting might have an easier transition.

What About the Controversy of an All-Meat Diet?

Even in what is arguably the simplest diet that ever existed, there's still some controversy. Among the topics that cause the most debate are organ meats, eating meat raw, and the superiority of pasture-finished meat. In the overall picture, these are minor issues when you compare them to the issues with just about any other standard diet. I'm certainly not discounting the idea that for certain individuals these variables can make a noticeable difference (either good or bad), but I don't see enough evidence to make a blanket recommendation for everyone.

Organ Meats

Organ meats are an extremely nutrient-dense source of food. It's unlikely that any other food can match organ meat like beef liver for overall nutrient density and bioavailability. If your nutrition is lacking, organ meat can be a tremendous tool for bringing you back up to speed. I don't see any major downside in adding organ meats to your diet. However, I also can't say that they are a must-have for all people at all times.

Many people point out that some traditional populations cherished organ meats and always ate "nose to tail." In many instances, organs were thought to have a special capacity for restoring health, so they were reserved for the infirm or older members of the group. Many cultures have elaborate recipes for these foods, which are considered to be delicacies. However, there were also societies in which organ meats, or offal, weren't considered desirable. They were cast aside or given to the poorer members of the population. So we can ask whether cultures that have historically used organs did so because of food scarcity or because they had a true desire to eat the organ meats for their health benefit. I think that question is open for debate.

Many people find organs to be unpalatable, and in the presence of enough other options, many forgo them. I can only guess what prehistoric humans might have done. If the organs were unpalatable to them and they had plenty of other meat, such as several thousand pounds of mammoth meat, would they have skipped out on the organs? If humans started by scavenging behind other predators, which is certainly plausible, then it's very likely they mostly had to make do with hindquarters and other scraps

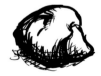

with some possibility that developing tools eventually enabled them to access marrow and perhaps animal brains to increase fat calories. This is a question that is likely impossible to answer.

I can tell you this, though: Many modern-day carnivores are getting healthy, reversing diseases, and thriving without eating any significant quantity of organ meats. The bottom line is that if you enjoy organs, you should have at them. If you've never tried them, you probably should see how you like them. If you don't find them pleasing and are in good health, I can't think of a great reason you should add them to your diet.

Raw Meat

Based upon the most reliable evidence we have, experts believe that humans began cooking around 400,000 years ago. Some people claim that we might have had control of fire as far back as 1.5 million years ago, but the evidence that supports that claim is not very robust. Also, we have fairly decent evidence that raw meat was still frequently consumed even after humans harnessed the power of fire. Even today, people in many parts of the world commonly eat raw meat. Dishes like beef carpaccio and steak tartare are served throughout the world, and sushi and sashimi also are popular. Among northern indigenous tribes, it's not uncommon for people to eat flesh directly off a freshly killed carcass. We shouldn't lose sight of the fact that during our evolution, eating raw meat was a reality, and we have an incredibly acidic stomach to cope with breaking down uncooked meat.

Does eating raw meat confer some special advantage? Certainly, some advocates of eating raw meat report easier digestion and lower requirements for food quantities because satiety with raw meat is better than with cooked. These people generally believe that their health is improved. You have to weigh these benefits against potential contamination risks. Those risks, while certainly real, are likely overstated, particularly if you pay close attention to sourcing.

Does raw meat provide access to more nutrition, or does cooking make it more accessible? I think this is a debatable topic, but let me state the obvious: If food is unpalatable to you, you will get precisely zero nutrition from it because you won't eat it. Aside from that, I know several people who've gone for long periods of eating raw meats, and they've noticed no benefits over cooked meats. Conversely, I'm aware of other people who state that raw meat is superior for them. I did a short trial of raw meat and found it to be more filling but not particularly palatable. That said, it does seem that many long-term carnivores find that over time they start preferring to eat meat that's less cooked. My conclusion is that you should decide what your preference is.

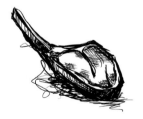

Grass-Finished Beef

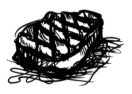

The most emotion-filled, contentious topic seems to be the controversy about choosing between grass-finished beef and conventionally raised beef. From a taste standpoint, it seems that what you are used to makes the biggest difference. Most of the beef in the United States is conventionally raised and finished for a short time on mixed forage and grain. This gives the beef a distinctive flavor and often produces a more significantly fat-marbled product that many prefer. People who are raised where a pasture-finishing technique is typically employed often state a preference for that flavor. I'm going to discuss more about environmental impact in a later chapter, but I will say that it isn't a very clear-cut black-and-white discussion.

What are some of the known nutritional differences in grass-finished beef compared to its grain-finished rival? On average, grass-finished beef tends to contain a slightly more favorable omega-3 to omega-6 fatty acid ratio because it's richer in omega-3. Omega-6 fatty acids are overconsumed in the standard American diet, and they probably contribute to some chronic health problems. People ingest the vast majority of omega-6 fatty acids via processed foods that contain high levels of omega-6-filled vegetable oils. The absolute amounts of omega-6 fats in either grass- or grain-finished beef is very low and is unlikely to be a problem, particularly when compared to other sources.

Another difference is that grass-finished beef has higher levels of CLA (conjugated linoleic acid) than grain-finished beef. CLA is believed to be beneficial in preventing metabolic syndrome and possibly has some anticarcinogenic properties. Grass-finished beef is also slightly higher in vitamin E and vitamin A content and has more alpha-linolenic acid.

The upshot is that grass-finished beef is certainly higher in several nutrients that may be considered beneficial. Does that confer a human health benefit? I'd say at this point the answer is no, or at least we don't know yet. In one of the few published human studies back in 2010, grass-finished hamburger, which tended to have a higher saturated fat–to–monounsaturated fat ratio, produced a slightly inferior result in HDL and triglyceride markers than grain-finished beef. However, that's just one study, and there's very little other data available. When we look at current carnivorous populations, there does not seem to be any difference in the efficacy of health improvement or disease mitigation between grass-finished beef and grain-finished beef. Certainly, some individuals say that they seem to feel better either on grain- or grass-finished products, but no clear pattern has emerged that enables me to give a blanket endorsement either way. I can only say that beef, regardless of finishing method, is a superior health food relative to just about any other food available.

There are lots of questions and differing opinions about the carnivore diet. The upshot is that you need to do what works for you. For some, this diet will not be a good approach. Some people are so metabolically tied to carbohydrates that they don't tolerate an abrupt transition, and ultimately it just might not be doable at all. If you have medical concerns or issues, involve your physician. Not all doctors will be supportive of this diet, although there are more and more doctors who are willing to empower their patients.

In the next chapter, I share some stories from people who've switched to the carnivore diet so you can find out how and why other people have worked this diet into their lives, and you can see that I'm not the only evangelist for this style of eating and its health benefits.

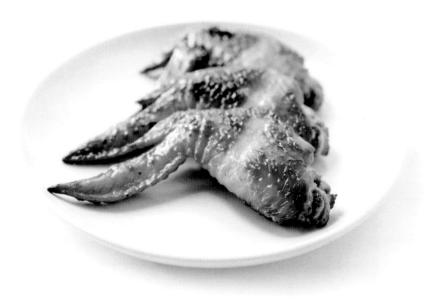

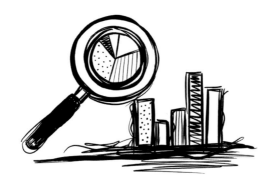

CHAPTER NINE

CHARACTER STUDIES **AND ANECDATA**

The entire reason for this book and the rise in popularity of this diet is because of the power of story. Let's face it; you can read study after study, learn all kinds of scientific facts, and memorize as much physiology as you want, but action often does not happen without inspiration. Reading or hearing the stories of people who have real-life experience with the carnivore diet and the benefits they've reaped while on it can be much more enlightening than all the scientific research in the world.

In this chapter, I describe four sample personas to summarize some of the characteristics and backgrounds of people who've gravitated toward the carnivore diet. Then I offer some anecdotes from real people who've agreed to let me share the compelling stories of their real-life struggles.

Persona Descriptions

Marketing teams sometimes come up with buyer personas, which are character descriptions of the person who may be the company's ideal customer. We could also call these "simulated people." I've created a few personas to illustrate ways in which people implement the diet and realize benefits from it. Although these stories are fictional, I've created them from composites of real people.

Big Jim

Jim was always a big guy. At the time he was fourteen years old, he weighed about 240 pounds. As a full-grown man at the height of 6'1", he wasn't profoundly obese, but he definitely was on the chunky side.

As he grew up, he played several sports and was a halfway decent outside guard on the high school football team. He even played for one season at a junior college. A knee injury when he was twenty ended Jim's football career, and his focus turned back to finishing school and starting work. He still periodically got motivated and headed to the gym.

Over the next two decades, Jim's health slowly got worse. The old knee injury started to act up more and more frequently. Ibuprofen became part of his routine. His diet was largely made up of fast foods—often greasy hamburgers, fried items, and a dessert. He was a big guy and had a big appetite. Jim's weight was pushing 340 pounds, and his coworkers knew him as a jovial guy.

At home, Jim was not quite so jovial. His wife, Barbara, had been concerned with his health for years, and she pleaded with him to see a doctor. Jim reluctantly agreed because, in all honesty, he felt pretty darn depressed, and his knee was getting worse.

During the medical exam, Dr. Miller quickly assessed Jim and determined his blood pressure was too high, and his BMI was 43. The doctor ordered several blood tests and referred Jim to an orthopedist to have his knee checked.

At the orthopedic office, Dr. Jones, who didn't mince words, said, "Look, you're just too darn heavy. You expect bicycle tires to support an airplane?" X-rays revealed some early arthritis, mostly on the medial, or inside, part of the knee. The doctor gave Jim a prescription for Mobic and told him to try it instead of the ibuprofen. The doctor also offered to prescribe physical therapy to strengthen the knee and told Jim to try to lose weight. The doctor requested that Jim come back in three months if he was still having pain.

Jim's follow-up appointment with Dr. Miller, the primary care physician, revealed that he had a moderately elevated total and LDL cholesterol, his triglycerides were high, he had some elevated markers of inflammation, and, according to his HbA1c reading, he was also prediabetic. At this point, Dr. Miller suggested that Jim would likely need to start some medications. However, because things were not yet severe, the doctor was willing to give Jim a chance to lose some weight and offered to send him to a dietitian. Jim agreed to try to work on losing weight because he didn't want to have to start taking medications.

At the dietitian's office, Jim was instructed to fill out a diet diary for a week and then return for a follow-up appointment. Upon his return, Sandy, the nice and seemingly fit dietitian, reviewed his diet, which Jim had fudged a bit. Even still, Sandy stated that Jim needed to make some fairly drastic changes. She designed a comprehensive plan of about 2,500 nutritionally balanced calories per day. Sandy discussed a plant-based diet with Jim, but he declined by stating that he liked meat too much and had never been a fan of vegetables.

At home, Barbara was on board for the new diet change because she also was holding onto about 30 extra pounds. Jim playfully complained about having to eat the "rabbit food" in the meals Barbara prepared, but he ultimately complied. After a few weeks had passed, Jim had lost about 11 pounds, and he was starting to feel a little bit better. After another few weeks, he had lost 18 pounds. Barbara was really happy with his progress, and some of Jim's coworkers had started to notice his weight loss.

During a follow-up trip to the dietitian, Sandy was pleased as she reviewed Jim's diet logs, and she encouraged him to keep going. Jim visited his doctor after a few more months had passed, and the doctor stated he was happy with the progress. However, he was considering prescribing medication for Jim because his labs were still a bit abnormal.

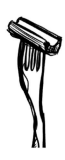

Jim doubled down in his resolve and tried to lose even more weight. He had been reading about intermittent fasting and started to incorporate it into his low-fat diet to ramp up the progress. He lasted only three days! At work, coworkers had a potluck birthday party. Jim carefully picked some carrots, celery, and a small amount of chicken and washed it down with a zero-calorie drink. He resisted the red velvet cake. At 3:00 p.m. that afternoon, however, Jim found himself back in the break room, and while no one was looking he devoured the remaining half of the cake. The sensation was magical; he was in absolute bliss because he'd been depriving himself for the past three months. He went back to his desk, feeling guilty but strangely satisfied.

Over the next few months, Jim started "cheating" more and more frequently. Pretty soon, Jim had gained back not only the 37 pounds that he'd lost but also an extra 5 pounds. Jim's wife Barbara was sad, but at the same time, she was secretly a little happy because she also didn't much like the diet. At the six-month checkup, Dr. Miller started Jim on a low-dose blood pressure medication, a cholesterol-lowering statin, metformin for his blood sugar, and an antidepressant.

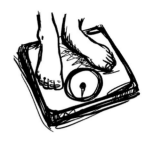

The orthopedist looked at the MRI of Jim's knee and suggested a knee arthroscopy to "clean up" his joint. Jim apprehensively agreed; three weeks later, he had a twenty-minute outpatient procedure. At the follow-up appointment, the orthopedist told Jim that his knee looked pretty beat up, but during the surgery he'd been able to remove most of the torn and loose tissues. Jim went to physical therapy for six weeks and then reported to the surgeon that the knee felt a lot better. Unfortunately, Jim was lying because he didn't want to hurt the good doctor's feelings. His knee was no better. To add insult to injury, he was just as fat as he ever had been, and he had recently started taking increased dosages of his high blood pressure medication and antidepressant.

At home, Jim and Barbara had grown increasingly distant. They rarely talked much, and most days ended with them falling asleep in front of the television. They hadn't had sex in well more than a year, and Jim didn't have any sex drive anyway. This pattern persisted for several years. Jim's weight increased to an all-time high of 384 pounds.

Convinced he wouldn't be around for many more years, and perhaps rightly so, Jim became increasingly withdrawn and apathetic. He no longer took pride in his work, and he rarely talked to his coworkers. The previously jovial and gregarious big guy had become a sad, oversized piece of the background.

Serendipitously, Jim saw an article that described some crazy people who ate an all-meat diet. Sure, the article wasn't in favor of the diet. It talked about how stupid the diet was and speculated that the only reason anyone had success with it was that the food was so boring that people tired of eating, so they lost weight. The article also pointed out that there weren't any long-term studies about the diet, and reams of evidence had proven that a person needed to eat fruits, vegetables, and whole grains and have plenty of fiber for long-term health.

However, by that point, Jim had started thinking that he wasn't that worried about long-term health. He hadn't enjoyed the other diets with all the vegetables and fiber, so he decided to try out the carnivore diet for one month. Barbara wasn't particularly thrilled, but she was at least a little happy that Jim was thinking about his health again. He went to the store and bought 60 pounds of meat. He also bought four dozen eggs, a few packs of bacon, and a carton of heavy cream.

The first few days were surprisingly easy: bacon and eggs for breakfast, lunch of a hamburger patty, and a dinner of steak. Jim was surprised that he didn't feel very hungry. By the fifth day, he was skipping breakfast, and he felt just fine. At the end of the first week, Jim had dropped 13 pounds. Even better, he had no hunger at all. However, things weren't perfect; he noticed that his energy seemed a little low, and he'd had only one bowel movement the entire time.

Jim started reading online success stories from people who'd followed a similar diet. He learned that supplementing electrolytes or drinking bone broth helped relieve low energy, so he tried it out. Although the difference wasn't huge, he did feel a little bit better. At work, he noticed he had a bit more energy, and he started to feel more like his old self.

After three months had passed, Jim had lost 44 pounds, and his knee pain had nearly disappeared. For the first time in many years, he had a positive outlook on life. He started to think about exercising, and both he and Barbara joined a local gym. Since starting the carnivore diet, Jim had remained pretty strict with the diet; he much preferred beef to other meats; he especially liked rib-eye steaks when he could get them on sale. For the first time in his life, he felt satisfied with his food. He had the willpower to resist foods that previously had been temptations. He'd had a few slipups along the way, and he'd noticed his gastrointestinal discomfort and knee pain had been worse at those times.

Jim visited Dr. Miller for a checkup after he'd been on the carnivore diet for six months. He'd lost 74 pounds from his highest weight, and his blood pressure had returned to normal. Jim talked to the doctor about going off the antidepressant and the metformin (the diabetes medication). Dr. Miller agreed to take Jim off his antidepressant, reduce the blood pressure medications, and reduce the metformin dosage. Dr. Miller asked Jim what he'd been doing to lose the weight. Jim explained the diet, and Dr. Miller said he didn't think following the diet long term was a good idea. He suggested that Jim consider adding fruits and vegetables. However, he admitted that the diet seemed to be working.

Jim was happy to get rid of some of his medications, and he and his wife Barbara celebrated with a date night, something they hadn't had in years. Jim tried to incorporate some fruits and vegetables in his diet, but he noticed that his stomach didn't do well with them. Furthermore, he didn't find them satisfying—particularly the vegetables. He went back to his normal diet of meat and eggs, with some cheese, fish, sausage, and bacon now and then. At his first anniversary of starting the carnivore diet, Jim's weight was down to 247 pounds, and he was the lightest he had been since his late teens.

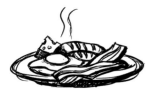

He had begun regularly exercising, and Barbara had lost 25 of the 30 pounds she wanted to lose. Both were genuinely amazed at how simple it had been. Jim's coworkers were amazed at his transformation and how much energy he had, but they routinely stated that they could never eat as needed to follow the carnivore diet. When he heard this, Jim just smiled to himself and thought about how easy it had been.

At the two-year point, Jim was off all medications; he had declined to remain on the statin drug despite Dr. Miller's concern. Jim felt the best he had felt in his entire life, and he had started experimenting with martial arts. He even considered getting into a health coaching job on the side. He and Barbara were as close as they'd ever been. For Jim, food was no longer the enemy, and he finally felt free!

Mindy Vegan

Mindy was 16 when she first started dieting. She'd never been fat, but she also hadn't been happy with her body. Her legs weren't shaped the way she liked, and she always wore long dresses to cover them. She tried all sorts of diets over the years and was constantly beating herself up every time she failed. By the time she was twenty-three, Mindy had been vegetarian for three years and vegan for a year and a half. When she first switched to a plant-based diet, some of her chronic skin problems started to clear up. She felt good to be helping the animals, and she tried to avoid any products that involved animals in the production process. Over time, though, she had started to notice some gastrointestinal issues, and her menstrual cycle was had become irregular.

Over the next several years, Mindy tried different variations of the vegan diet. For example, she attempted to go raw vegan for about three months, but she noted increasing problems with her stomach. She saw her doctor, who suggested some probiotics and talked to her about possibly including some animal products in her diet because her lab work indicated she was anemic.

Mindy politely declined to incorporate animal products into her diet because, at this point, she was very passionate about not harming animals. The thought of eating meat again was repulsive to her. She tried some juice cleanses and experimented with various enemas recommended by some vegan experts who shared their work online. Each month she spent more money on supplements in the hope that she'd feel a bit better, and it became increasingly difficult to find vegan foods that didn't bother her digestion. Mindy, who was 5'4", had lost quite a bit of weight; she was down to 103 pounds. Her physician diagnosed her with clinical depression and hypothyroidism; she also was constantly tired. She took several medications and an increasing number of supplements. She often did not want to leave her house, and she spent most of her days on the computer arguing with people about the virtues of veganism. The sicker she got, the more she clung to her beliefs about vegetarianism and veganism. Mindy's mother came to visit, and she couldn't believe how frail her daughter had become. Mindy's mom insisted Mindy stop her vegan diet and tried to help by going to the store and cooking some eggs for her to eat. Her mother's attempts to "help" infuriated Mindy; she screamed at her mother, told her how much she hated her, and demanded that she get out of her house!

Over the next six months, Mindy became more and more negative in her interactions with people in her online community. She even began to advocate for violence against people who ate or produced meat. After an episode of intractable vomiting that led to severe dehydration, she checked herself into a hospital. She weighed only 94 pounds. The doctors at the hospital rehydrated her via intravenous fluids and controlled her vomiting with medications.

Alone, sad, and broken, Mindy knew the decision that she needed to make. On her way home from the hospital, she bought a carton of eggs and some breaded fish sticks. She started to cry, and she apologized to the animals. Mindy spent fifteen minutes looking at a fish stick through tear-filled eyes before she could muster the courage to take a bite. She choked and coughed and continued to cry. By the fourth bite, she became ravenous and quickly finished off the rest. Then she made four eggs, which she also greedily ate. For the first time in years, her body felt as if it was getting nourishment. Her stomach did not hurt at all, and she didn't have any painful bloating. Over the next several weeks, Mindy continued to eat this way without tears, even though she still felt sad for the animals.

At first, she kept the fact that she was no longer vegan from her vegan friends because she feared the repercussions that she knew would surely come. Because she'd recently been such a vocal supporter of animal rights, she had a hard time wrapping her head around the fact that she had "failed" as a vegan. She quietly distanced herself from the vegan crowd and told a few people that she just couldn't do it anymore because of how sick she'd gotten. A few people criticized her, but the overall reaction wasn't that bad. In fact, a few vegans even wished her well and hoped she got better. Mindy said that she hoped that she could go back to being a vegan someday. Inside, however, she knew that she never could go back to it.

Over the next six months, Mindy's weight bounced back to 107 pounds. She felt much better, and she started dabbling in the carnivore diet. The more she listened to her body, the more it asked her for meat. In fact, she even started craving raw meat at times. She started finding herself drawn to organ meats, realizing that the extra nutrition provided by them was energizing her. Her teeth, which had deteriorated during her days of high fruit raw veganism, were slowly getting better. Her mood brightened, and she got back in contact with her mother. After a tearful reunion, Mindy began to realize just how badly her vegan heroes had misled her. She became angry at them and started publicly speaking out against them both in her personal life and online.

One year after transitioning fully to the carnivore diet, Mindy felt the best she had since early childhood. Her digestive issues had cleared up completely, and the dry skin and cold hands she always had as a vegan were gone. She had started exercising and had recently begun strength training. Her weight was up to 112 pounds, and for the first time in her life, she began to feel comfortable with her body. Although she still wanted to make some improvements, she was no longer embarrassed by who she was. At this point, Mindy was eating about 1.5 pounds of meat each day; most of her calories were coming from red meat, fish, eggs, and the occasional piece of organ meat. After two years on the diet, Mindy was as happy as she had ever been, and she had recently been able to reintroduce a few nonanimal products to her diet—mainly berries and a few bits of starch here and there. Mindy had finally found her comfort zone!

Nurse Elaine

By the time she was forty-seven, Elaine had raised three children, had spent twenty-two years in the nursing field, and recently had been through a divorce. Over time, her weight had slowly crept up, especially since her third child had been born. She had been diagnosed with fibromyalgia, and she'd been on antidepressants for the last three years (with limited success). As someone who worked in the medical field, she was aware that many of the physicians she had worked with regarded fibromyalgia as a disease of the mind; they didn't consider it a "real disease."

After her divorce, Elaine gained 26 pounds. She was 5'6", and her weight hovered around 185 pounds. She had tried numerous diets over the years and had always had temporary success, but she'd gained and lost the same 20 pounds dozens of times. As a nurse, she was well aware of the risks created by added body weight. She was particularly concerned about breast cancer because she had lost her older sister to the disease a few years prior, and she'd also had an aunt who had succumbed to it.

Elaine had been a nurse so long that she was on autopilot at work. She still enjoyed patient care, but as a senior nurse, many of her duties were administrative. She calculated that she could retire after seven more years of work, and she looked forward to traveling and reading her books of classic European literature.

Her fibromyalgia was never severe enough to keep her from work, but there were days when she didn't feel very well. Unfortunately, the bad days had begun to occur with greater frequency. To make matters worse, she was entering the early stages of menopause. Although she had already raised her children, she was somewhat sad to see her fertility leave her. Elaine also knew that more weight gain often came with menopause, which was a prospect she was not looking forward to.

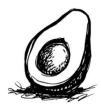

On her forty-eighth birthday, Elaine decided to try out the ketogenic diet that she'd heard about. Several of the nurses on her shift had been successful in losing weight on it; unfortunately, all but two of them had gained back most of the weight. The biggest challenge was that the nurses station was a constant collection point for chocolates, baked goods, and donuts that the patient's families brought in to say thank you for the care the nurses provided. Elaine was generally pretty good at avoiding these dietary booby traps, but she often found that her willpower would wane during her menstrual cycle or when she felt stressed.

As Elaine embarked on the keto diet, she purchased several cookbooks and eagerly looked forward to trying out some of the delicious-looking recipes. Friends with experience on the diet told her not to go crazy on eating the desserts too often, and she liked the fact that she could eat plenty of vegetables because she had always known that the best way to get healthy included plenty of salads. Surprisingly, she was able to stick to the diet without much trouble. What friends had told her about the lack of hunger was turning out to be true.

After three months on the keto diet, Elaine had managed to drop 32 pounds. She was at the lightest weight she'd been in well over a decade. Her fibromyalgia symptoms were still present, but the severity was less. Her doctor was able to cut the dosage of the antidepressant in half. She was really enjoying the keto diet.

When she first started, she had been very meticulous about tracking her macronutrient ratios; she endeavored to keep her fat at around 80 percent and her net carbs lower than 20 grams daily. She checked her blood ketone levels several times a day. She knew to limit her protein so that she would not be driven out of ketosis, and she generally stuck with white meats and fish. She began to get comfortable with baking with alternative ingredients like almond flour and coconut flour, and she had plenty of stevia in the cupboard. As an occasional treat, she would enjoy a couple of squares of dark chocolate, and she began to enjoy the 85 percent cacao variety. A few times per week, she would treat herself to a fat bomb. She drank her coffee with heavy cream, butter, or even MCT oil.

Eventually, Elaine's weight loss stalled, and her occasional dark chocolate treats were becoming more and more frequent. She started to grow tired of all the baking, and she no longer was as strict with her macros. She'd stopped checking ketones a long while ago. She had been on the keto diet for just a little less than two years. She was still pretty good at not cheating on the diet, but she just wasn't where she wanted to be. For a few months, she tried to add more carbohydrates in the hope that she could jump-start her metabolism or at least help out her hormones. At this point, she was in the middle of menopause. Although her symptoms were not as bad as some of her friends had described, it was not completely smooth sailing.

Elaine's brief foray into including more carbohydrates didn't go very well; she gained 6 pounds in one week, and her fibromyalgia pain worsened. She was frustrated, but she went back to her keto diet and resigned herself to thinking that it was as good as it could get. One day when she was looking for recipes on a ketogenic support group website, she came across someone talking about how they were having success on an all-meat diet. At first, she thought the idea was preposterous, but she clicked a link the person had included, and she soon discovered a group of thousands of people who were participating in this bizarre diet. She was shocked to learn that many group members were women, and several claimed to have gotten rid of depression and lost weight. A few even specifically said that their fibromyalgia had drastically improved. There were even people who mentioned that ailments like psoriasis and rheumatoid arthritis had gone away. Elaine made a mental note of that detail because one of her nieces had been struggling with psoriasis for the last several years, and it had recently been getting worse despite treatment with increasing amounts of medications.

Elaine spent the next three months exploring websites about the carnivore diet, and she became fascinated by some of the stories she was seeing. She didn't understand how changing the diet to only meat could lead to getting healthier. She knew a small minority of people had severe food allergies and gluten intolerances, but the reasons for people's interest in the diet seemed to go way beyond that. She noticed that many of the members of this group had come from a ketogenic background and were talking about how much better they felt once they let go of the vegetables and the artificial sweeteners.

Three weeks shy of her fiftieth birthday, Elaine decided to try this wacky all-meat, carnivore diet for one month. She was able to get some grass-finished steaks from her local grocery store, and she bought some eggs and a small bit of heavy cream to put in her coffee; she had no intention of quitting coffee at this time. She had gotten some sea salt to use on her steaks and bought some grass-fed ghee to cook with. The first day was a struggle. Elaine's ex-husband had been the grill master in the family, so she didn't have much experience with cooking steaks. She thought it was too chewy. The next few days were similar, although she did allow herself to eat some cheese. While she was at work, she ordered some bunless burgers, which came in a lettuce wrap, from the cafeteria. She felt a bit guilty for not eating her usual big salad, but she also had noticed that she wasn't experiencing as much bloating as normal. In the first week, she lost 4 pounds, and she had noticed that her fibromyalgia symptoms were basically gone.

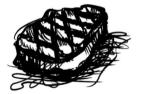

By the end of the month, she had adapted to the diet and was starting to look forward to her meals. She became more comfortable with preparing steaks and was enjoying the lack of calculating and planning. Because she was doing well, she decided to give it an extra month. At the end of the second month, Elaine observed that her symptoms of menopause were hardly noticeable, and for the first time in a while, she was sleeping well at night. Her appetite began to pick up, and what she had previously thought were unexciting, bland foods suddenly became very appetizing. She started to crave steaks. As she began to eat more, her weight started creeping up. Initially, she was concerned by this, but she was feeling so good otherwise that she didn't want to change her diet. Elaine's coworkers started to call her "the lion lady."

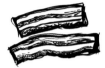

After six months on the carnivore diet, Elaine was off all her medications, and she felt pretty good. The one problem was that she had gained 23 pounds over those six months. She told herself that some of the weight gain was probably due to increased muscle, but she also could see the unmistakable extra layer of fat on her thighs and belly. She started to ask some other people about their experiences, and Elaine found out that this weight gain wasn't uncommon. It seemed to be especially typical among women, particularly those who had lost quite a bit of weight before starting the carnivore diet. She received advice that ranged from, "Just give it time; eventually, your body will finish healing, and then you'll lose the weight," to, "You need to eat less and start to exercise."

Elaine had spent her entire life doing the eat-less-and-exercise-more thing, so she wasn't keen to start doing it again, particularly considering how good she felt. At her next physician visit, Elaine's doctor didn't see any abnormalities in Elaine's lab data. In fact, the doctor was quite surprised by how good things looked considering Elaine's diet.

After another three months had gone by, Elaine's weight had stabilized. She had lost about 3 pounds since the six-month point. She was still heavier than she had been at her lowest weight on the keto diet, but considering that her fibromyalgia was gone and her depression had not come back, she took it as an overall win.

Eventually, she did cut back just slightly on her food intake. At first, she had to make a conscious effort to stop eating just before she reached the point of full satiety. After a month or two, Elaine found that her appetite was naturally slightly less. She started to exercise, but it wasn't an activity she enjoyed, so she abandoned it in favor of reading some of her favorite books while sitting in front of her fireplace.

After two years on the carnivore diet, Elaine's weight had gone down even more, but it was still about 5 pounds more than her lowest ketogenic diet weight. At this point, she was completely fine with where she was. She found that as long as she remained about 90 percent strict on her diet, her depression and fibromyalgia symptoms stayed away or would be minimal, and her weight was stable.

CrossFit Keith

Keith, who was thirty-two years old and 5'10", had been training for seventeen years. His undergraduate degree in kinesiology served him well as a strength and conditioning coach. For the past four years, he had worked with a variety of clients including overweight stay-at-home parents, retired executives, and high-level athletes. He kept up with the latest literature and constantly updated his programming to reflect any new knowledge he gained. It was a lot of hard work and long hours. He often started at 5:00 a.m. to meet with his clients before they went to work, and on some days he ended his workday after 9:00 p.m.

In addition to his busy coaching practice, Keith was an avid CrossFit athlete, and he'd done fairly well in competitions over the last few years. He'd just missed qualifying for regionals two years before. Unfortunately, a shoulder injury had put a damper on his recent training. Keith was still a lean and muscular figure at 185 pounds. He had almost the perfect build for the varying demands of CrossFit.

On most days he was able to train twice a day, often working with his training partner, Ty. The two would push each other to their limits, and the friendly rivalry was a great driver of success. Keith's shoulder issue was caused by a small labral tear that most affected him when he was doing overhead lifts, like the snatch, and in some of the gymnastic moves, like muscle-ups. Although he still performed the movements fairly well, he always felt a small amount of apprehension, and his shoulder commonly ached for a few days afterward. Mobility exercises had helped somewhat, and he frequently did rehab exercises on his shoulder. Keith found that he was relying on over-the-counter anti-inflammatory medications more and more frequently, although he typically was reluctant to take them. When he saw an orthopedist about the issue, the doctor had discussed a possible surgery if things did not improve with rehab.

Keith had always relied on a higher carbohydrate approach to fuel his workouts, and he was well aware of the literature that supported that style of eating during an intense performance such as CrossFit. He religiously fueled his workouts with a pre-workout drink and was diligent about having a mixture of carbohydrates and protein immediately after his workouts. He had been aware of a few members of his CrossFit box who had talked about a ketogenic diet. None of them were particularly high-level athletes, although Keith had observed that several of them had leaned out and improved their performance a bit. However, he was skeptical. He had read numerous studies that had shown that a ketogenic diet might be effective for high-level performance in ultra-endurance sports, but it didn't appear to be effective for glycolytic activities like CrossFit.

Unfortunately, a year later, Keith's shoulder was no better, and he ended up having the surgery. A forty-five-minute outpatient arthroscopy had

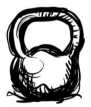

revealed a small tear in the posterior aspect of his shoulder's labrum. Two anchors held the labrum in place, and the doctor told Keith that his recovery would likely take about six months. Keith diligently did his rehab, but at the end of the six months he was still having some pain, he had lost a little bit of mobility in the shoulder, and his attempts to return to training were frustrating.

For the first time in his life, Keith was starting to get soft. He didn't like having fat hanging around his gut, so he embarked on a diet to lean out. He knew to keep his protein consumption up and slowly walked down his calories, and he gave himself a regular "refeed day" every week or so. He knew this strategy had worked well for his clients in the past, and, after some time, he started to lean out. Because he couldn't train like he wanted to, he also couldn't eat as much as he typically did. He didn't particularly like this situation, and although his gut had shrunk, he also was a lot weaker than he wanted to be.

Keith's work schedule was just as demanding as ever, and he and his wife had just welcomed their first baby into the family. Keith became increasingly tired and found his motivation to train was waning. Also, his desire to constantly track his calories and macro percentages fell by the wayside. His chronic shoulder pain, the stress of a new baby, and his busy coaching practice had him conceding that his days of athletic competition were coming to an end.

One day, Keith's client Sergio mentioned that he was doing the carnivore diet and was having great results. Keith smiled to himself and thought, "What a dumbass." But over the next few months, he saw that Sergio was starting to get lean, and his performance was getting quite good. Jokingly he asked Sergio if he was still doing "that crazy all-meat thing." Sergio replied, "Yes, indeed," and said that he was feeling the best he ever had.

Keith did some online research about the carnivore diet. He found some articles stating that it was a bad idea and that it was a sure way to end up with a heart attack or colon cancer. He also read some anecdotal accounts from people who claimed to have been cured of all sorts of medical problems. Keith knew anecdotes were not a particularly great source of evidence because they were often unreliable. However, it seemed unusual that there was such a high frequency of reports from people who'd had joint pain go away. After thinking about it for a few days, Keith decided that he would try it for one week.

Keith decided that if he were going to try the diet, he would do it the best way he knew how. He understood that a potential nutrient deficiency could be an issue, and also he wanted to eat only grass-finished beef. He diligently included some liver, wild-caught salmon, pastured eggs, and a variety of cuts of beef. He told his wife about his crazy experiment and explained that he was doing it for only one week. She was used to his crazy training, so she shrugged her shoulders and said, "No, thanks."

After three days, Keith's shoulder pain was almost completely gone. When he was between clients at the gym, he'd do a few clean and jerks with just 135 pounds on the bar, and he felt no pain. He began to think that maybe there was something to this wacky diet. Over the next few days, Keith felt pretty well other than having a few carbohydrate cravings and a mild headache. When the week ended, Keith dove into a big bowl of oatmeal topped with raspberries, cinnamon, and a small amount of brown sugar. The next day, his shoulder pain was back. After a few more days of continued pain, he decided to try the carnivore thing again, but this time he planned to do it for a whole month.

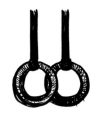

Twelve days into the second attempt, he was back to training. He also noticed that his sex drive, which had always been decent, was ticking up a notch. He felt fairly energized and started seeing some forward progress with his lifting. At the end of the month, he was feeling as good as he could remember, at least for the last several years. He noticed that his abs were starting to become visible again, and his wife noticed that he seemed to be in a better mood. His sleep was still a bit choppy because the baby would wake up once or twice in the middle of the night, but that was getting better as she got older. Despite the sleep interruptions, Keith generally felt well rested and was able to get through the day without any problem. He decided to keep going.

Up to this point, Keith had mainly been focusing on strength work and polishing his technique, particularly with the Olympic lifts and some of the gymnastic movements common to CrossFit. He started to ramp up some of the metabolic conditioning workouts and noticed that he was struggling. He had read enough to know that people can build strength and muscle without carbohydrates, and he had been able to put on about 5 pounds of lean mass over eight weeks, even though he was visibly leaner. His problem with the metabolic conditioning persisted; he couldn't do what he needed to do without the carbohydrates. He started to incorporate some fast-digesting carbohydrates near his training times, and he noticed an immediate improvement. His shoulder flared up a few times, but the issues were fairly mild.

Over the next six months, Keith began surpassing his previous bests in his strength numbers. He hit a 35-pound personal best in the deadlift, pulling 555 pounds. He also nailed a 280-pound snatch. His time on Fran, a benchmark Workout of the Day that includes thrusters and pull-ups, went from a previous best of 2 minutes, 25 seconds down to 2 minutes, 14 seconds.

Over time, Keith's need to supplement carbs before workouts became less necessary; he began doing a large percentage of his workouts completely without them. He would save his carbohydrates for select workouts and during competitions. His training partner Ty was impressed by his performance and wanted to know his secret. Keith showed him a picture of a steak and laughed. That year, Keith qualified for CrossFit regionals for the first time.

Anecdotes

People write me all the time to tell me how they've struggled with health and weight issues for years; tried all kinds of medical and nutritional therapies to effect change; and followed their doctors' orders in the hope that they'd see improvement in the quality of their lives only to end up disappointed, frustrated, and still unhealthy. Then, when they learn of the carnivore diet and decide to give it a try, things start to turn around, and they can't wait to tell other people about it. The anecdotes I've included here are just a tiny sample of those stories.

> " The thing I've noticed is when the anecdotes and the data disagree, the anecdotes are usually right. There is something wrong with the way you are measuring it. —Jeff Bezos

Charlene

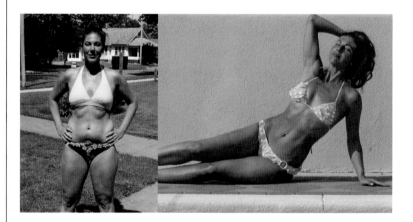

People often ask my husband, Joe, and me, "What made you decide to do the carnivore diet more than 20 years ago?" In a nutshell, this is what I tell those people who ask:

Back in 1998, after years of countless health issues throughout my childhood and adulthood (including Lyme disease), trial and error with foods led us to a diet of only fatty red meat and spring water. That's what worked. Period.

Here is a list of some of the most important changes I experienced:

- **Amenorrhea:** My ten-year bout with missing periods cleared up as soon as I used animal fat as my only fat source. I ovulated within days and had a period two weeks later. Since changing my diet, I've been perfectly regular, and I've had two healthy pregnancies and deliveries.

- **Trichotillomania (pulling out my eyelashes and eyebrows):** I developed this disorder when I was 8, and it lasted through adulthood. It ended about a month after I started my meat-only diet.

- **Paralysis:** This was one of my worst symptoms by far. An attack would include numbness, starting with my hands and feet, that worked slowly toward my torso until I was in overall body shutdown. These attacks would last for hours or days. It took about a year to reverse completely.

- **Debilitating fatigue:** I was exhausted to the point of falling asleep while I was at work or driving a car. This symptom also took about one year to reverse.

- **Muscle twitches:** I would have more than 100 twitches in one minute. I noticed an immediate improvement in this symptom, but a year passed before it completely reversed.

- **Depression:** Before I changed my diet, I suffered from relentless darkness and suicidal thoughts. I didn't know how I'd get through the next hour, let alone the whole day. Fortunately, the depression lifted rather quickly—probably in less than a couple of weeks.

- **Degenerative disc disease and sciatic nerve pain:** The discomfort from these issues dissipated within a couple of months.

- **Excess weight:** Over a few months, I lost about 50 pounds.

- **Rage:** One of the effects of Lyme disease is a personality change. I experienced episodes of rage, which became shorter and less intense until they vanished after a few months on the carnivore diet.

- **Extreme allergies/sensitivities to pollens, chemicals, and foods:** I had a nearly immediate reversal in my allergies.

- **Eyesight:** Within about a month and a half, I no longer needed contacts or glasses.

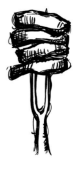

The following symptoms, which are less severe in comparison to the previous list, took a month or less to reverse. Some even resolved in days.

- Brain fog and mental confusion. My once-sharp mind could barely keep up with a conversation.

- Cyst-like acne on my face, neck, shoulders, back, and chest.

- Eczema on my hands, neck, and face. At times, the condition was like second-degree burns on the backs of both my hands. I couldn't curl my hands at all.

- Bloating and chronic gas that doubled me over in pain.

- Indigestion and acid reflux.

- Restless leg (more like restless body).

- Bingeing and purging.

- Headaches and migraines.

- Edema.

- Heart pains and irregular heartbeat.

- Halitosis.

- Terrible tinnitus.

- Constant white spots on my tonsils.

- Dry, flaky scalp and skin.

- Purple fingers in winter or when stressed.

- Inability to handle cold or heat.

- Susceptibility to colds and especially flu.

The moment Joe and I realized that diet could change everything, it finally gave me the power to try, to fail, to retry, and eventually to win! There is life after illness. That I *know*!

Chris D.

I'm forty-five years old, and the carnivore diet has saved and completely transformed my life! At the time of writing, I have lost more than 220 pounds and reversed all my serious health conditions.

Even though I was in the health and wellness industry (as an herbalist and licensed massage therapist) for 25 years, my health continued to deteriorate, and I gained more and more weight, eventually tipping the scales at more than 500 pounds. I was diabetic and hypertensive, suffered from gout and kidney stones, and experienced daily pain. I struggled with serious diverticulitis (pain, frequent infections, need for antibiotics and hospital visits) for years, and it eventually led to a perforated colon. I spent a week in the hospital, and I was very nearly septic and could have died. Doctors told me that inevitably I would need surgery to remove all or part of my colon.

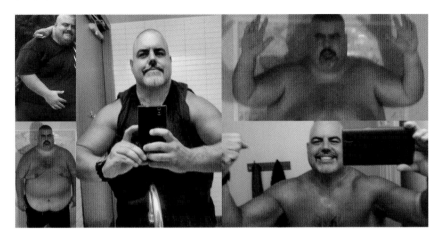

I tried every diet under the sun and used all manner of pills, potions, and lotions—anything that I thought could help. I spent thousands of dollars on supplements and alternative therapies. I was vegetarian for a time, and I tried several radical eating plans, including meal replacement shakes and extended fasting. I even spent a few months eating only baby food. *Nothing* worked. I became more and more disabled and depressed. I was unable to walk across a room without being short of breath. I was hopeless that things would ever change. I closed my eyes in bed every night, not knowing if they would open again. A CPAP machine kept me breathing, but I knew that my heart and other body systems could not go on much longer like this.

Toward the end of 2018, I began following a strict ketogenic diet. I lost a little weight and saw some improvement in my health, but most of my conditions persisted. Then I began reading stories of people who experienced dramatic health improvements, including with some of the issues I had, by following the carnivore diet. I decided I had nothing to lose, and on December 1, 2018, I went carnivore and removed all plants and fiber from my diet. My health transformation since then has been nothing short of miraculous! My weight started to melt off. My energy and mood improved. And my diverticulitis, diabetes, kidney stones, gout, leg edema, ocular migraines, prostate issues, and other issues completely resolved. *I haven't had a single symptom of any of them ever again.*

I am off *all* my prescription medications and daily supplements. I eat meat when I'm hungry and drink water when I'm thirsty. I don't count calories, macros, or anything else. I love the simplicity and freedom that this way of eating brings. Without any fiber in my diet, I experience perfect digestion and elimination. My energy and mood are consistently high, and a lifetime struggle with anxiety and depression is all but gone. I am the healthiest, happiest, and strongest I've been in my life.

In the past, I missed out on many things with my family because I wasn't able to join them for most activities; for example, I couldn't fit in the booth in restaurants or the seats of amusement park rides. Now I can fully participate and enjoy life! I can walk anywhere, and I hike with my children in the mountains near my home. I feel like there is nothing I can't do. I even won almost $3,000 in an online weight loss contest I entered. And I was able to make these improvements without feeling deprived or like I was "on a diet." I don't struggle with hunger or cravings. Rather, I am well-fueled and satisfied with the most nutrient-dense, delicious food on the planet.

The carnivore diet has given me my life back as well as giving me a new purpose to help people struggling just as I was. With my new-found health and energy, I became certified as a health coach and hypnotherapist. It's now my passion to help other people regain their lives through the carnivore diet and other lifestyle changes. There is hope!

Laura

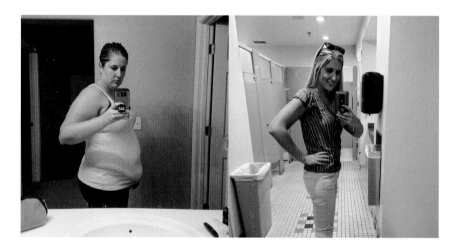

In my adult life, I've never had two consecutive birthdays on which I've weighed the same. The past ten years have been a roller coaster of gaining and losing large amounts of weight. The only way I knew how to lose weight was with restriction. I was good at being restrictive so that I got results, but long-term restriction was never sustainable for me because I was constantly hungry.

One year, I even tried a vegan diet and had mild success. I lost 50 pounds, but the majority of my hair fell out. The vegan diet left me with low energy, and I was very nutrient deficient. Coming off of that diet, I gained back all the weight I'd lost plus more. I found success with traditional low-carb and keto diets at first, but like other diets, I was never able to be consistent and refrain from "cheating" because I felt so deprived. Through all the "diets" I tried, I still held onto my same terrible relationship with food. I had just replaced my old food habits with "keto" versions of those bad foods. And I still dealt with constant mindless eating.

In February 2018, I had knee surgery for a torn meniscus. My knees couldn't handle the weight that I was carrying around. In March 2018, I had to get on the scale at a follow-up doctor appointment. I'm 5′8″, and I weighed 263 pounds. I was considered prediabetic. I weighed more that day than I weighed the day I went into labor with my son, who was two at the time of that appointment. I felt overwhelmed, so I started yet another low-carb crash diet. Within days, I was already planning a cheat day to reward myself. I was eating processed protein bars, lots of veggies, and a small amount of meat. I felt the same deprivation I always had before, and, once again, my hair began to fall out.

A couple of months later, I learned about the carnivore diet. I thought the idea that people don't need vegetables was insane. I had dealt with constipation and hemorrhoids for many years, and I believed that eating foods with massive amounts of fiber was the only way to have a healthy digestive system. However, I gave eating only meat a try for a week, and I had my first pain-free bowel movement in years. At the end of the week, I had a big salad, thinking there would be nothing bad in that. I spent the weekend dealing with bloating, cramps, and intense digestive issues. My body was telling me that the veggies were causing the issue. Problems in my body that I'd thought were just normal issues were flaring up after I'd eaten that salad.

At that point, I researched more about the carnivore diet, listened to Dr. Shawn Baker's podcast, and consumed any information I could find! I began a strict carnivore diet and told myself it would be a trial. The longer I ate only meat, the better I felt. I soon realized that my acne and skin issues, which I thought were normal for me, had cleared up. My digestive system had never been healthier. Most shockingly, the cheat meals I had planned were less tempting because I had no cravings. Eating meat naturally made my body want to fast. I started out eating three meals a day, but I found that I was no longer hungry for breakfast. I also found that with a large lunch of steaks, I wasn't hungry for another meal later. I settled into a one-meal-per-day routine and ate around 1.5 pounds of steak, typically rib-eye. The weight continued to melt away, and I had never felt more satisfied. The need for cheat meals was completely gone because I didn't feel any restriction. I had struggled with anxiety for years, which was another thing I thought was a normal part of my personality, and I saw tremendous improvement in that area as well.

By October 2018, I had lost 100 pounds. My energy had increased, and my hair began to grow back thicker than before. I continued to follow a strict carnivore diet through the holidays, and by the end of January 2019, I had lost 120 pounds total. I also started going to the gym around this time; I've been lifting weights two to three times a week. I've been maintaining a weight of about 140 pounds since January, but my body is continuing to change as I get stronger. At times I've felt the pressure to add variety to my diet, such as other meats and eggs. Each time I try to move away from steak, though, I begin to feel anxiety and cravings, and I'm less satisfied. It's strange how the perceived restriction of eating only steak has given me so much freedom from my addictive food tendencies, emotional eating, and anxiety.

The rest of my family has transitioned to this lifestyle. My husband has his own amazing carnivore success story (see page 153). Our children eat a high-protein diet, free from sugars, grains, and seed oils. They're learning that too much sugar makes us sick, and we need lots of protein and fat to be healthy. They receive conflicting information at school when the Food Pyramid comes up, and the teachers say we all need lots of whole grains and vegetables. They happily educate their teachers that grains are unhealthy, and kids don't need to drink milk. I'm proud to raise them with a better understanding of nutrition than I had and to help them create healthy relationships with food.

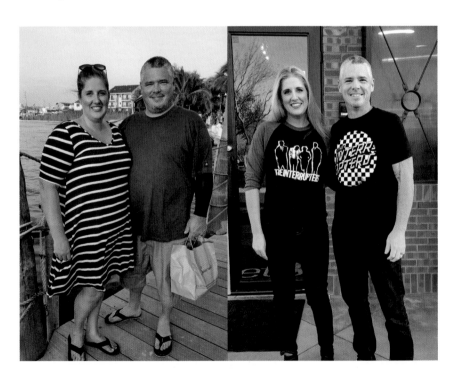

Chris S.

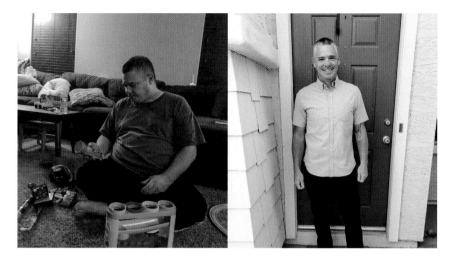

I graduated from high school in 1993 and decided to join the U.S. Air Force. When I saw the recruiter, he told me that I had to lose some weight to be accepted. I was eighteen years old and weighed 245 pounds; I needed to get down to 185 pounds before I left for basic training. I got to work, and after six months of chicken, rice, and running, I had lost 60 pounds and was ready to go. Four years later, I finished my service and jumped right back into the bad habits that would eventually almost take my life.

On Christmas morning 2016, instead of opening presents with my family, I drove myself to urgent care to get checked out. I'd had a serious fever the night before, and a large red spot on my elbow was growing rapidly. I had an infection that developed into necrotizing fasciitis (flesh-eating disease). I nearly didn't make it, but after numerous surgeries and seven weeks in the hospital, I came home changed forever. It took me some time to recover and sort through the trauma. Eventually, I concluded that what almost took my life was my poor health. Two years prior, after fifteen years of eating a garbage diet, I had been diagnosed with type 2 diabetes. I took the medications prescribed, but I didn't take the disease too seriously, so I continued with a lifestyle that eventually caught up to me.

In early 2018, I weighed 294 pounds. I had type 2 diabetes, hypertension, sleep apnea, daily headaches, and bouts with anxiety and depression. I was taking many medications several times a day, and I slept with a CPAP machine. I researched strategies I could use to get healthy and started my journey that April. I began with the ketogenic diet combined with intermittent fasting because there seemed to be a lot of people having success using these tools. Immediately my weight began to drop, and I felt better daily.

We've always been taught to eat plenty of fruits and vegetables for optimal health, and I believed what I'd learned, of course. That's what the doctors, teachers, and parents told us, so it had to be true, right? The truth is, I always hated eating plants (unless they'd been processed and refined), but I still forced myself to eat some broccoli with my steaks. I felt pressure because of what I had learned, as well as because my family was watching what I ate.

Then I came across some folks who were eating the carnivore diet. Immediately I thought, "This is for me!" I watched Dr. Shawn Baker, a vocal proponent of the carnivore way of eating, on *The Joe Rogan Experience*. Dr. Baker's approach was simple and logical. After going down the rabbit hole of information online, I was on board. Plants were gone, and I was truly happy with what I was eating for each meal. Even during the days when I was eating "trash," my favorite food was always a good steak. Now I was able to eat that every day and feel good about it.

My weight dropped rapidly, and my energy level increased. I was getting better day by day. After I lost about 80 pounds, I found the energy to get into the gym. I began a resistance training regimen that had me gaining strength and muscle mass while I was losing fat. After eight months of the carnivore diet, my weight was 178 pounds (a 116-pound loss). At forty-four, I feel better than I have in my entire life—even better than when I was a teenager. I also have more energy and vitality, and I'm stronger and sharper.

I saw my doctor in April 2018. At that time, my HbA1C was 11.6, and my blood pressure was 140/90 (although I was on medication). When I went back in December 2018, the doctor hadn't seen me in eight months. In the intervening months, I had stopped all medications within a few weeks of being on the carnivore diet. My blood sugar was good, so I stopped the metformin and glyburide. My blood pressure dropped dangerously low, so I stopped taking Lisinopril. I did some research on the statin medication, and then I dropped it. I no longer needed my CPAP machine. I had no more headaches or pain, so I didn't take NSAIDs. I was medication-free for the first time in my adult life. My blood work came back in December 2018, and I had an HbA1C of 4.9. My fasted insulin was 4, and my C-peptide was 1.8. I was no longer insulin resistant, and my fatty liver had cleared up. Needless to say, my doctor was shocked but pleased. He added, "diabetes – resolved" to my medical record. Of course, my LDL was high, so the conventional training meant he recommended that I take a statin, but *my* indicator for my need for medication is how I feel, and I feel great.

Today I continue to maintain weight loss, work out daily, and live my best life with the support of my family. We try to teach our children the importance of proper nutrition and an animal-based, species-appropriate diet. I had to go through some rough times and severe trauma to wake up, but I am happy to be awake and reaping the benefits in so many ways.

Sylvia

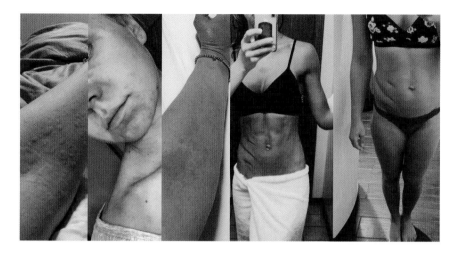

I started experimenting with different diets back in high school. At that point, I was mostly trying to improve my athletic performance. Later, in college, I decided to go vegan after watching a couple of terrifying vegan documentaries. It didn't take long for me to shift toward the vegan diet because I didn't want to take part in any of the animal suffering that was portrayed in those documentaries. I thought I was going to save the world by not eating animal foods. I went from a whole food, low-carb, Atkins-style diet to vegan, and my health started declining very quickly. It took four years of eating a raw vegan diet, of which one year was purely fruitarian, to deplete my body to a point where my digestion got really bad, and my body started reacting to healthy foods like green vegetables with red, itchy rashes. Also, after a year of the fruitarian diet, I started dealing with severe depression and binge eating, which later turned into a six-year-long battle with bulimia.

Eventually, my health declined to the point that I had no choice but to start eating animal products again. It took me a while to convince myself that eating animals is the right thing to do. It didn't help that many of my vegan friends and vegan leaders kept telling me that I wasn't doing the diet the right way and that I wasn't supplementing with the right things. Trust me; I did a lot of research because I wanted the vegan diet to work for me.

Finally, after learning that the plant-based lifestyle creates more harm than good, I decided to break from the vegan lifestyle by buying some fish. After my first nonvegan meal of wild-caught fish, my mood changed drastically, and my depression lifted almost immediately. Later, I switched to more of a ketogenic diet, which included small servings of animal protein. I felt pretty good for a few months as I followed that lifestyle, but after going through three surgeries to clean up necrotizing fasciitis, my gut and digestion was a mess again. The only foods that I didn't react to were meats.

I heard Dr. Shawn Baker talk about the carnivore diet on a podcast and decided to give it a 30-day trial. That was more than a year ago. I've been living exclusively on meat, and my body just keeps improving and healing—better body composition, healthier hair and nails, improved libido, better vision, and drastic changes in my mental health. I've never felt so calm as consistently as I do now—no more mood swings. Also, the carnivore diet got rid of my six-year-long eating disorder, which had almost ended my life.

It took some time to find the right types of meat, experimentation with removing eggs and dairy, and trial and error to find the right amount of food that made my body thrive on a daily basis. With time, I became more in tune with my body, and now I'm able to eat to satiety and stop eating when I'm not hungry.

Not needing to count calories or track macros has been very freeing for me. Some people may view the carnivore diet as very restrictive, but I've never felt freer than I feel right now. I'll continue with the carnivore lifestyle as long as it keeps serving my health and well-being. How long will that be? We shall see.

Erik

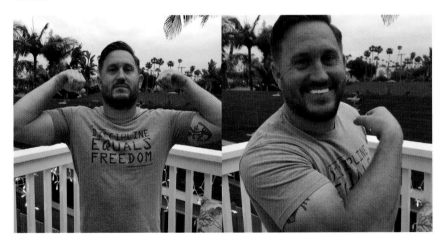

I've been approximately 90 percent carnivore for the last nine months, and my life has only improved since switching to the carnivore diet. Every aspect of my life has improved since I made the change to an all-meat diet.

I'll never forget the first time I came across the subreddit r\zerocarb. I read the description of the group and laughed when I saw the part about not eating any plants. I vividly remember telling myself, "These people are full of it. Everyone knows we need to get nutrients and fiber from plants." This kicked off a nine-month investigation into what being healthy means.

For reference, I'm an engineer by profession, so I tend to try to read everything about a subject.

For me, the carnivore lifestyle has been a massive journey in expanding my understanding of the world and what conventional science has taught us. It has also taught me a lot about how humans fit into the circle of life. We all have learned about the Food Pyramid. It's been one hell of a journey just unlearning what is good and healthy for us. A year ago, I never would have thought that giving up plants would benefit me.

I'm fortunate that I haven't had any major health issues in my life. One thing that has troubled me was irritable bowel syndrome. I also frequently got up to urinate in the night. Those are the main issues I had in my twenties. One cause for the nighttime bathroom visits probably was excessive alcohol use, but I attribute the IBS to my diet. Once I switched to the carnivore diet, the symptoms disappeared within a week. I honestly could not remember the last time I slept through the entire night without waking up to use the bathroom.

The other issue I'd experienced was allergies, and the second major benefit to the carnivore lifestyle was that they went away! I'd always had a problem with an itchy throat, and I was able to breathe only through one nostril at a time. Within three weeks, my allergies were gone, and I could breathe normally.

I also have spondylosis from an injury I sustained when I was twenty-two. Since then, I've suffered from chronic lower back pain. I've played sports my entire life, and I'm specifically into wrestling. Over the fifteen years I wrestled, I developed inflammation in my acromioclavicular joint (the joint at the top of my shoulder). Since going carnivore, my shoulder pain has completely gone away, and my back pain has reduced about 90 percent. Sometimes I get sciatica, but since I've implemented yoga with my carnivore lifestyle, my joints and back feel great!

I've been playing sports, working out, and generally taking an interest in health my entire life. Since moving to the carnivore diet, I've noticed my endurance while running has increased dramatically. I'm able to work out longer, and my strength has significantly increased! If I miss a few days of working out, I don't lose strength or body composition like I used to. Another benefit that I hadn't anticipated is that the more I eat like a carnivore, the more focused on life I become—both professionally and personally.

I believe we're on the brink of a health revolution. The more this lifestyle grows, the more I've seen propaganda for veganism grow. It's been very interesting to watch developments in both areas over the last few years. My goal is to help Dr. Baker on the research and analytical side of the carnivore movement. I can't help but think about what we have left to unlearn about nutrition, physical health, and mental health. We've been fed so much BS all these years.

The single biggest benefit of my switch to the carnivore lifestyle hasn't been physical. The best benefit is that it's opened my mind to endless possibilities on how to improve my life. It's changed the way I view our economy. It's changed my life by helping me focus on locally sourced food, and I've picked up hunting as a sport. Because I've adopted the carnivore lifestyle, I've learned how destructive monocropping is to the land and how beneficial it is for ruminants to graze that same land instead.

Another important aspect of the carnivore lifestyle is that it's taught me how easy it can be to fall prey to "group think." There's a huge push right now from people who want to blame part of the global warming problem on "cow farts," when in fact cow farts have an insignificant effect on our environment. Just think for a moment how many resources it takes to get fruit from one end of the globe to the other and what kind of effect *that* has on our environment. The carnivore lifestyle has helped me think for myself, listen to my body, and improve the lives of my loved ones.

Nicole

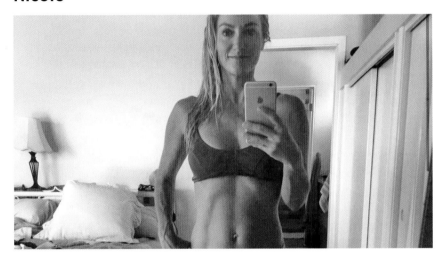

When I was about eighteen, I decided to give up all meat, egg, and dairy products. I believed it was a good thing for my body and the environment. Before making this decision, I had eaten the standard American diet, which included a fair amount of processed foods, sugar, and alcohol.

During my first few years on the vegan diet, I felt very good. I lost some weight and was happy with my decision. However, when I was about twenty-three, I started to have some issues with endometriosis and irregular periods. A few years later, I started to struggle with my energy level; I was in a constant state of fatigue. I tried adding vitamins B12 and D and iron to my routine, but I still was extremely tired. I had my vitamin D levels tested, and they were very low despite the supplementation. I experienced gallstones and pancreatitis, which led to having my gallbladder removed. I also was experiencing depression and anxiety around this time, but I didn't associate those issues with my diet.

Since I wasn't feeling well, I decided to escalate my diet to a raw food vegan diet. I thought this must be what I needed to do to feel better. I believed that by eating only raw plants, I would get the most nutrients possible. I ate only uncooked fruits, vegetables, and sprouted nuts and seeds. Everything I ate was either organic or grown at home. Unfortunately, my health steadily declined. I began to get sick repeatedly with flulike symptoms, and my anxiety and insomnia became more intense. I was constantly cold, and I had systemic candida that I could not get rid of. The fatigue became overwhelming. My hair began falling out, and my stomach constantly hurt. I was chronically constipated, yet I persevered through my vegan diet. I could not fathom that it was causing my issues. I continued this way for a few more years, despite encouragement from doctors to add meat into my diet. I tried acupuncture, naturopathic medicine, homeopathy, reiki, chiropractic, and standard Western medical doctors. It wasn't until several more years had passed that I shifted to more of a plant-based diet, adding in some yogurt, eggs, and fish. I did see improvements, but only a few.

In 2012, a doctor diagnosed me with ulcerative colitis, a painful autoimmune disease that causes pain in the intestines, bloody stools, and fatigue. I had a very seriously damaged gut lining. I shifted my focus to doing whatever I needed to heal this disease in particular. I tried going back to both a vegan diet and a raw vegan diet, but the symptoms became worse with each of those diets. I removed all root vegetables and legumes when I tried a low-glycemic diet; I had some positive results, but the colitis symptoms were still there, even if they were less significant. I explored all kinds of other diets: macrobiotic, low FODMAP, nightshade-free, GAPS, Paleo, and ketogenic. I did get some relief on the ketogenic diet; however, at that point, I was still eating a good amount of plant materials—a lot of almonds and very little ruminant animal meats. I continued on the ketogenic diet for one year, but I would still have some symptoms of colitis, and I was gaining weight.

In May of 2018, I began the carnivore diet, eating only beef, lamb, fish, chicken, eggs, and some bacon. My symptoms were reduced greatly, and within about four months, every symptom I had was gone. Even the problems I'd had that were separate from the colitis had been resolved. I no longer had insomnia. I no longer had thyroid issues. My hair stopped falling out and grew thick and long. My sex drive was stronger than ever, and my cycles involved almost no PMS. I felt calmer, happier, and less stressed than at any time in many years. I finally got relief from years of struggling once I had eliminated *all* plant food from my diet. It was a miraculous change that even I was shocked to see.

As I write this, I have been on a zero-carb carnivore diet for one year, and I continue to thrive and get stronger. I share my message with anyone who wants to learn. I was so fixated on a dogma of fruits and vegetables being the cornerstone of health that it seemed impossible that I could be free of health problems by eliminating them. I'm forever grateful to those who spoke out to help spread the word, especially Dr. Shawn Baker, who has been a major inspiration. He has shared experience, knowledge, and science that proves meat is healthy. Meat heals.

Brett

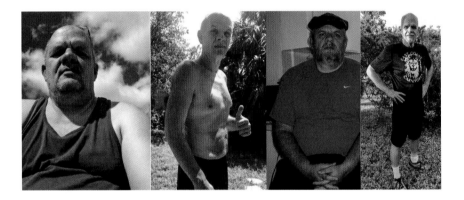

A doctor first diagnosed me with major depression in 1990. In 1995, I started taking antidepressants per my doctor's order. Thus began the cycle of wellness versus illness that gradually turned into my being ill most of the time.

For me, depression manifested as extreme dissatisfaction with everything and everyone, especially myself, and it often presented as anger. There was a huge component of sadness underneath this dissatisfaction. I looked like I was furious even when I believed I was in a pretty good mood and having a good day.

The depression altered, warped, and twisted everything I heard, saw, touched, felt, and thought, and nothing was ever in my favor. If my wife expressed something positive with joy in her voice, I heard the words, but I registered her tone of voice as dark and despairing as if she was suggesting something was amiss. Because I loved my wife (still do!) I would ask, "What's wrong?" She naturally would be puzzled and ask what I meant, and an argument would almost invariably ensue because we couldn't communicate with each other. It created horrible levels of tension and anger in our marriage.

In 2007, I had a textbook nervous breakdown. Crippling insomnia and anxiety joined the party.

My doctor put me on much stronger meds that included Effexor, Wellbutrin, Ambien, Remeron, Lamictal, Abilify, Seroquel, Ativan, Trazodone, Latuda, Symbyax, and many more! From 1995 until the end of 2017, my brain chemistry was constantly under assault by these medicines that never really helped me for more than a few weeks.

By January 2015, my psychiatrist recommended I either undergo electroconvulsive therapy or commit to long-term hospitalization. I weighed 289 pounds, and I wasn't sure whether I would survive the year because my depression was so serious. I thought about suicide more often than I would admit, even though I had no real desire to end my life. The illness relentlessly brought the notion to the forefront of my thoughts.

Later that year, I discovered I could treat my depression symptoms successfully with cannabis. Cannabis allowed me to perceive myself more realistically, and I realized I had become very overweight. Having had success with some weight loss some years earlier on a modified Atkins diet, I began a low-carbohydrate, high-fat diet and started walking daily. By the end of 2015, I was off the antidepressants. By the end of 2016, I was off the Ativan (after eight years of daily prescribed use). By the end of 2017, I was off the insomnia meds.

But I was still dependent on cannabis. I live in Florida, and even as a legal patient, cannabis is very expensive. I hated being dependent upon it to treat my mood. Then I discovered a clip of Dr. Jordan Peterson on Joe Rogan's podcast as he talked about the carnivore way of eating, and then I found Rogan's interview with Dr. Shawn Baker!

There was a chance I could eliminate my depression by eating meat and drinking water? Count me in!

On July 16, 2018, I began living carnivorously. I have only consumed meat and water from that day.

Ten days into the experience, all my joint pain was gone. Beginning on day 23, I felt the depression vanish. I am 100 percent free of depression now! No more mood crashes! No more ranting and raging! I was free.

My anxiety problem gradually has improved each day. Now, at more than ten months in, I have no anxiety issues to speak of.

My skin, which used to be very dry, cracked, and peeling, has cleared up immensely. Skin tags have disappeared. My quality of sleep has improved dramatically. I frequently get seven to eight hours of sleep.

The background noise in my head is all gone. My ability to observe has improved immensely.

Every aspect of my life has improved since I began eating meat and drinking water. I'm fifty-eight, and I'm on no pharmaceutical medications. I'm thriving, and so is my marriage! I not only have a life, but I look to the future with great optimism. This is why I'm a thankful carnivore now and forever!

Dawn

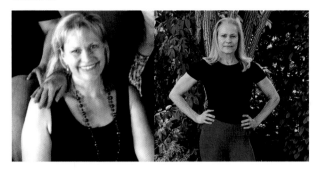

I've struggled with several medical problems for many years—some for my entire life. I have hypermobile Ehlers-Danlos syndrome (hEDS, an inherited connective tissue disorder), postural orthostatic tachycardia syndrome (POTS), osteoarthritis (OA), Hashimoto's thyroiditis, and other autoimmune disorders. I've spent far too much of my life sick, in bed, and in pain, particularly in the past fifteen years. I started needing NSAIDs regularly when I was in my thirties, and at times, I've needed stronger medication because of the frequent injuries associated with hEDS.

When I woke up in the morning, the first sensation I experienced was pain. One or both of my shoulders, my hip, and my ankle would be completely or partially dislocated every morning. I would spend several minutes reducing my joints, just to be able to get out of bed. Throughout the day, I would dislocate or partially dislocate my joints many times. My shoulders were eventually completely unstable. I could no longer raise my arms without having a shoulder dislocation or subluxation, which made routine tasks, such as brushing my hair or dressing, very difficult. I knew that I would soon need bilateral shoulder stabilization surgery.

To make matters worse, I was about 30 pounds overweight. For a person with joint hypermobility, being overweight is especially problematic because it increases joint pain, instability, and frequency of injuries. As happens to most patients with chronic pain and illness, I was fatigued, I slept poorly, and I suffered from some degree of depression. Unfortunately for hEDS patients, doctors say that there is no solution, and we can only expect to get increasingly worse. Before I changed to a carnivore diet, this was certainly my experience.

In June 2018, I read a short article about two people who experienced improvement in their chronic health problems by eating a meat-only diet. Frankly, I thought it sounded crazy. I'm generally skeptical of fad diets, and I dislike the diet industry in general. I abhor claims of miracle cures or the latest superfood. As a physician, I am rooted in science and evidence-based medicine. As a person with multiple medical problems, I needed a solution. I decided to do a little research on the carnivore diet. I came across Dr. Shawn Baker's articles and listened to his podcast, *Human Performance Outliers*. I found it intriguing and decided to try the carnivore diet for thirty days as an experiment. I knew enough about diet to know that simply reducing my carbohydrate intake would be helpful with weight loss. Beyond that, I had no expectations. This decision turned out to have been one of the best decisions I've ever made.

I began to notice the changes in my body within a few weeks. I started losing weight after about two weeks, which I expected. What I did not expect was the noticeable reduction in joint pain and an overall increase in my energy level. I decided the improvement was enough that I would continue for another thirty days. My weight loss continued steadily, and my pain began to improve gradually. I was able to begin working out. I noticed that I was getting stronger far more quickly than I anticipated, particularly for my age (at that time, I was fifty-seven) and relative state of health. By the second month, I had fewer joint dislocations and subluxations. My shoulders, hip, and ankle stopped dislocating. By the end of the second month, I no longer woke up with multiple joint dislocations, and pain was no longer the first sensation I experienced. Overall, I felt better. I knew I was onto something and decided to stay with it.

After nearly a year on the carnivore diet, I continue to improve. I've lost about thirty pounds of fat, and I've gained a considerable amount of muscle. I haven't had a full joint dislocation in about ten months, which is a lifetime record for me. My arthritic joints are less painful, and I have improved range of motion in those joints. I sleep better than I have in many years. The low-level depression I experienced is gone. I have better mental focus and clarity. Activities of daily living are much easier for me. I can brush my hair or reach over my head without pain or joint dislocation. I kneel or squat without pain and get up without help. My pain level is perhaps 5 to 10 percent of what it was. I no longer take any pain medication. These developments are nothing less than remarkable. I've had improvements in my other health problems as well; I haven't had any autoimmune flare-ups, and my POTS symptoms are far better controlled than they once were. I've been able to reduce my thyroid medication to one-third of my previous dose, and my thyroid labs are normal.

I admit to not having an explanation for many of the improvements I've had in my overall health after changing to a carnivore diet. As a physician, I look forward to learning more about research on this way of eating. For the time being, I'm merely grateful to have discovered this unexpected solution to many of my considerable health problems. My only regret is that I didn't discover the carnivore diet about thirty years ago. I very likely could have avoided much of the pain and suffering I've endured.

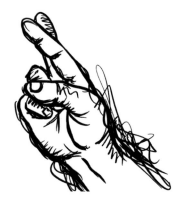

CHAPTER TEN

VEGANISM: THE FALSE HOPE

"Carnists are triggered and worried. They know their way of life of eating animal flesh will end soon. They feel threatened. It's just a matter of time before all people on the planet will be vegan. Carnism is not sustainable. We activists target children, teaching them the loving ways of veganism and an all-plant diet. Eventually, laws that are fueled by vegan activism will be enacted to make it illegal to kill animals for food. New generations will come into power, armed with vegan knowledge to change the landscape. The few carnist holdouts will have no choice but to go vegan or face prison and even death. You will discover it's wonderful, healthy, and compassionate. Carnism will soon be a thing of the past. There is nothing to fear."

—An example of a vegan comment from one of my YouTube videos

In the last few years, we've seen increasing popularity in vegan, vegetarian, and other plant-based diets. Celebrities, vegan physicians, and other influencers have popularized these diets. These people contend that plant-based eating plans are better than diets that include meat because they're healthier, they're better for the environment, and they result in less animal suffering. Sounds like a winning plan! It's not surprising that many people, particularly younger individuals, have started to adopt these diets. We should all have the freedom to choose to eat in a way that best supports our health and conforms to our ethics. Much of the world does not have that luxury.

In this chapter, I discuss why a vegan diet may not deliver what it is billed to offer, and I counter some of the common talking points. We have been subjected to an unrelenting and one-sided message for far too long, and now, with the support of processed food companies (which benefit from an anti-meat message), the noise about plant-based eating has gotten significantly louder.

The Push for Plant-Based Diets

Are we being "forced" to adopt a plant-based diet? Almost daily, we see an ever-growing media campaign that demonizes meat and seems intent on guilting us into not eating it. Unfortunately, as I pointed out earlier, when we eliminate animal food, we don't replace it with kale and broccoli; instead, we eat more processed garbage. That's just how it goes, and the processed food companies, which have incredibly deep pockets, are well aware of this. In a recent paper, Marco Springmann and his collaborators stated that a meat tax is a necessity to save lives. Springmann is a vegan, and the journal in which he published his article *(PLOS ONE)* was founded by Patrick Brown, the CEO of Impossible Foods, which is a company that manufactures plant-based "meat." If that's not a conflict of interest, I don't know what is.

Very recently, a three-year collaboration effort called the EAT-Lancet Commission on Food, Planet, Health has made its way into the headlines. The commission, which has a supposed goal of saving the world, is acting as a springboard to drive worldwide guidelines on how we should eat.

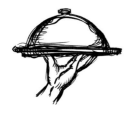

The fact that it has been spearheaded by vegan activists who parade as scientists and is heavily funded by processed food companies, pharmaceutical companies, and the "plant-based" wife of a billionaire hotel mogul is evident in the commission's final report. The report encourages a diet that allows for just 7 grams of beef per day and features 53 percent of an individual's calories coming from sugar, grains, and processed seed and other vegetable oils. This recommendation is basically a recipe for copious amounts of cheap processed foods with the barest amount of animal nutrition needed to prevent outright malnutrition. The poor suckers living in developing countries will likely be forced to eat this garbage because they're often subject to corrupt governments and have little opportunity to complain.

When it comes to wealthy developed countries, the EAT-Lancet Commission acknowledges that the population will not willingly accept this style of diet, so the plan is to start imposing draconian taxes and other restrictive legislation or trade agreements to more or less force citizens' compliance. For those people who will proclaim, "They'll have to pry that rib-eye from my cold dead hands," guess what? No one will have to pry anything. Instead, purchasing meat will become prohibitively expensive, so there will be nothing to pry out of your hands. Honestly, the people who are most likely to suffer will be the younger generations because they're being systematically brainwashed to accept that humans don't need to eat animals, and it's normal to eat processed foods and live on supplements and pills. Make no mistake, despite all the vegans yapping about their "whole-food plant-based" diets, the anti-meat agenda is ultimately about getting more and more people to live on processed foods.

When we start critically examining some of the claims vegan diet advocates make, we see that they often are misleading—in my view, sometimes deliberately so. As I've gotten more involved with nutrition over the last few years, I've noticed the alarming and ever-growing number of vegan disaster health stories. I started a Facebook group called the Restoration Health Vegan Recovery Group, and within just a few months, well more than 1,000 members had joined. I regularly see accounts of wrecked gastrointestinal function, depression, anxiety, skin and dental problems, and a whole lot more. Although many vegan evangelists will say, "Those people just didn't do it correctly," most of the these recovering vegans were adhering to the teachings of leading medical doctors who are proponents of the vegan, whole-food lifestyle, and they were taking appropriate supplements. The good news is that many of these folks see a significant improvement in their health after they add animal products back to their diets.

Regarding the supposed health advantage of a vegan diet, the most popular argument infers that diet determines longevity and references epidemiology studies and the "Blue Zones," which are areas of the world in which the population lives to an average older age than in other parts of the world. As I pointed out earlier in the book, that epidemiology is critically flawed because correlation does not necessarily equal causation. However, vegan advocates continually rely on these types of studies to claim that plant-based diets are superior for yielding positive health outcomes.

For example, the people who live in Blue Zones are often homogeneous groups genetically. They live in favorable climates with low levels of pollution. They have low smoking rates, access to good health services, and a culture that prizes the elderly. One of the often-cited Blue Zone groups is the population of Loma Linda, California, which is largely comprised of members of the Seventh-day Adventist Church, a group that generally lives a long time and includes many vegetarians. Some details that advocates typically gloss over include that this population has extremely low rates of smoking and alcohol and coffee consumption. They tend to get more exercise than the general population and to be better off financially. They have a strong social support system. When you look beyond the basic facts, it's interesting to note that even in this group, the longest-lived subgroup is people who include animal protein (in this case, fish) in their diets.

Another comparable population in the United States is the Mormons (the Church of Jesus Christ of Latter-day Saints), who have similar health and lifestyle practices but do not promote a vegetarian diet. Guess what? The Mormons live just as long as the residents of Loma Linda!

The Okinawans are another Blue Zone population that is often held up as a poster child for a plant-based diet. It has been supposed that Okinawans had a high plant-intake diet, and at one time they had a very long life expectancy. However, the assumption that they ate little meat has been seriously challenged. Okinawa has been called the "island of pork," and many of their traditional dishes are heavy in pork products. The data that proclaimed Okinawa a "Plant-Based Paradise" was based primarily on a 1949 survey, which was shortly after the island had been devastated by World War II, and the pig population had been decimated. Before the war, the island was estimated to have 130,000 pigs, but during the war, that number dwindled to around 7,000 animals. At the time of the survey in 1949, the citizens of post-WWII Okinawa were eating what amounted to a starvation diet, which wasn't reflective of their usual pork-heavy diet. By the mid-1950s, the island's pig population had recovered, and the residents resumed eating their porkalicious diet. Okinawans typically ate about 50 percent more pork than their Japanese neighbors and consumed far less rice and grain. A study of the Okinawan centenarians noted that none of the individuals were vegetarian.

If we want to continue to play the epidemiology game, then we can look to modern Hong Kong, where the citizens are prodigious consumers of meat and also enjoy what is arguably the longest life expectancy on Earth.

I'm not saying this correlation necessarily proves that meat equals longevity (because lots of other factors determine how long someone lives), but it sure as heck makes it hard to say meat is life-shortening.

Researchers have conducted several formal epidemiological studies over the last few years, and those studies indicate there's no advantage to a plant-based diet when it comes to mortality. These include the 45-and-up study from Australia, which had a sample group of 250,000 people; the Epic Oxford study, which included 60,000 people; and the European-based PURE study, which was the largest study ever with more than 135,000 participants. As I said, these studies are epidemiological, and you need to take them with a grain of salt, but they clearly run counter to what vegan advocates suggest.

Let's look at the population of India, where people consume the least amount of meat per capita of any nation on the planet but have astonishingly high rates of both cardiovascular disease and diabetes. Other interesting anecdotal data is that India is last in the world per capita for the number of Olympic medals won, and it has recently been noted to have the highest mental health disease burden in the world. As with any scenario, many factors contribute to the situation, but an overall inferior nutritional strategy probably plays a significant part. Many vegan critics would say that the citizens of India are mostly vegetarian rather than vegan, and they would blame the population's health problems on dairy. However, if we look at the top dairy-consuming countries in the world, which are in Scandinavia, we find a generally long-lived and relatively healthy population.

Something more important than the epidemiology studies is the fact that people who eat a meat-based diet don't eat junk food, smoke, or drink, and they do get exercise and generally take care of themselves; they're very healthy. There are plenty of folks who eat a plant-based diet but are obese and sick, and often they're eating the same garbage that the fat, sick meat eaters are eating. Processed carbohydrates, refined vegetable oils, and sugar make you sick regardless of whether you include meat in your diet. Americans now consume as much soybean oil as they do beef, and overall beef consumption has dropped by about 30 percent since the 1970s. (See Figure 10.1.) One of the reasons some people have some success with whole-food, plant-based diets is because they're eliminating processed carbohydrates, sugars, and oils, not because they're omitting meat.

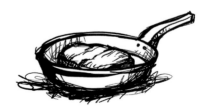

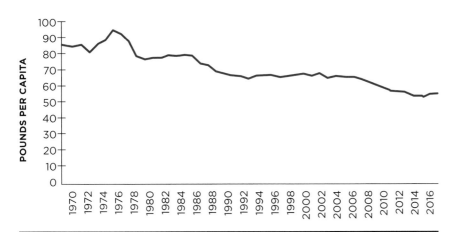

U.S. Beef Consumption
1970-2017

Figure 10.1
Per capita beef con-
sumption in the U.S.,
1970–2017 (data sources:
USDA ERS and WASDE)

Almost any diet is an improvement over the standard American diet. The problem with plant-based diets is that many people develop significant medical issues over the long term, particularly if they're not careful with meal planning and aggressive supplementation. A fairly recent study from the Humane Research Council showed that 84 percent of people who adopted a plant-based diet ultimately gave it up, typically within a few months and often for health reasons. For some people, pursuing a vegetarian or vegan diet isn't about health; it's about ethics. I've heard many vegan proponents admit that they would never include meat in their diets even if its absence was damaging to their health. I find that kind of blind commitment to be a sign of a mental health disorder, but, of course, adults are free to choose what they feed themselves. At this point, organizations in several countries have issued cautionary statements concerning the nutritional adequacy of vegan diets for children.

In the United States, approximately 70 percent of our caloric consumption derives from plant-based sources, most of which are grains, vegetable oils, and sugar-based foods. Further removal of animal nutrition doesn't lead more people to eat kale; instead, they seek out other forms of concentrated calories, such as vegetable oils, sugars, and refined grains. Our health has only worsened as our consumption of animal products has declined since the 1970s. The processed food manufacturers know that people consume more processed food when they don't eat animal products, so those companies are on board with the plant-based movement. I believe that they use vegan activists as unwitting shills to steer more people toward their low-nutrition, high-profit products.

The dramatic rise in vegetable oil consumption (see Figure 10.2) is a typical example of how processed alternatives replace animal products. A meat-based diet has the exact opposite effect, resulting in a large reduction of processed food intake, and the media engages in massive pushback because their advertisers bid them to. Registered dietitians are trotted out in the media to decry the horrors of eating meat, as if humans hadn't been eating it for centuries. However, these days people are starting to mistrust people in the nutrition industry because that profession has failed us. We are only getting sicker, and the continued platitudes about balance and moderation are basically an admission of cluelessness. I've yet to be made aware of any wild animal that is required to eat a "balanced diet" to be healthy.

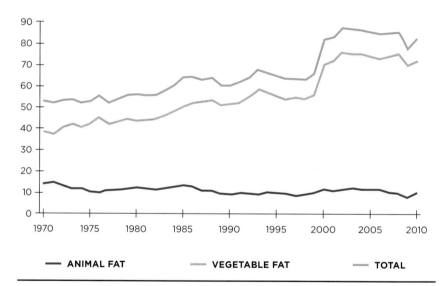

Pounds per person per year (fat-content basis)

Figure 10.2
Fat and oil consumption between 1970 and 2010 (source: USDA)

Environmental Issues

The environment is another area in which the data spewed forth from highly biased activists has made an impact. Currently, some people seem to think that forgoing meat is the greatest possible thing one can do to protect the environment. We see the media, whose motivation is influenced by advertisers, increasingly repeating this BS propaganda.

Let me talk a little bit about greenhouse gases. *Cowspiracy: The Sustainability Secret*, a popular vegan-friendly documentary, claims that animal agriculture creates 51 percent of worldwide greenhouse gases. This claim circulated for several years, and many people still reference it as gospel.

In 2006, the Food and Agriculture Organization (FAO) of the United Nations proffered a study, *Livestock's Long Shadow*, which proposes the calculation that animal agriculture accounts for 18 percent of worldwide greenhouse gases rather than the previously reported 51 percent. This number was significantly less, but there was a problem with the data. The FAO did a "life cycle assessment" on animal agriculture, which means that they tabulated every molecule of methane, carbon dioxide, and nitrous oxide that went into producing 1 kilogram of meat and added those numbers to the direct methane emissions from the cow. The resulting figure included food, water, transportation, processing, packaging, and so on from the birth of a calf all the way until the piece of steak made it onto a plate. The FAO compared the gases produced during the whole production cycle only to what comes out of a car's tailpipe. An apples-to-apples comparison would require an analysis of the production of the car, all the required materials, and the fuel; the transportation involved in supplying the materials; the maintenance of roads; and so on.

Professor Frank Mitloehner from the University of California at Davis made the authors of the study aware of the severe error they'd made, and the authors of *Livestock's Long Shadow* conceded that point; they issued a revised figure that was even lower: 14 percent. The vegan documentary *Cowspiracy* used the incorrect higher estimate. If we compare direct emissions among all industries, then the worldwide production from animal agriculture is a mere 5 percent of the total. That number isn't insignificant, but it's certainly not the primary driver of climate change, as the vegans and the fake meat/processed food companies would have you believe.

The numbers used in the FAO report are worldwide numbers, and it's essential to understand what that means when it comes to those of us in the United States and other developed Western nations where the pressure to move to a plant-based diet is most prevalent. If we look at current United States greenhouse gas emission as compiled by the U.S. Environmental Protection Agency (EPA), we see that all animal agriculture accounts for less than 4 percent of total greenhouse gas emissions, and beef cattle account for only about 1.9 percent. (See Figure 10.3.) To put this in perspective, Professor Mitloehner has determined that if every single person in the United States went vegan, and every animal that we eat magically vanished, the global effect on greenhouse gas emissions would decrease by approximately 0.3 percent.

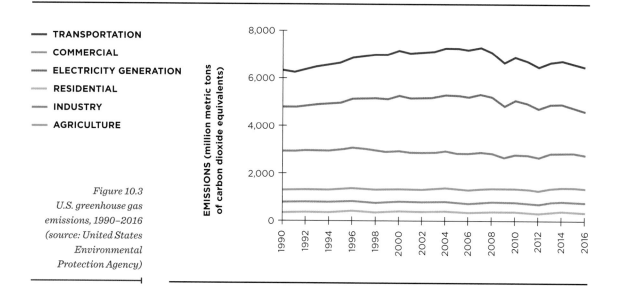

TRANSPORTATION
COMMERCIAL
ELECTRICITY GENERATION
RESIDENTIAL
INDUSTRY
AGRICULTURE

EMISSIONS (million metric tons of carbon dioxide equivalents)

Figure 10.3
U.S. greenhouse gas
emissions, 1990–2016
(source: United States
Environmental
Protection Agency)

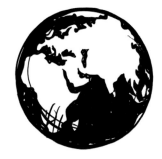

Then why are the worldwide numbers higher? Well, for one thing, the United States puts out a hell of a lot of greenhouse gases; the country leads the world in per capita greenhouse gas production. China takes the prize for the largest total amount, but because of that country's tremendous population advantage, 1.3 billion, their per capita number is less than the United States' number. The 14 percent worldwide calculation from the FAO includes much of the world that's still relatively undeveloped; therefore, the vast majority of greenhouse gas emissions from undeveloped countries comes from animals. In fact, if we were to roll back the clock 100 years or so, we would find that at that time, there was a much higher worldwide contribution of greenhouse gases from animals than we see today because our use of fossil fuels has dramatically increased over that time. In North America, vast herds of bison roamed across our plains and numbered between 30 and 60 million for centuries before Europeans arrived on the continent. The current cattle population in the United States isn't much higher than that. Also, it's important to note that since the 1970s, greenhouse gas emissions from cattle in the United States have dramatically *decreased.* This reduction is due to several factors involving increased efficiencies and a lower total number of animals. It's also important to note that none of these numbers take into account the positive impact that well-managed cattle have on improving soil and sequestering carbon in the ground, the potential of which is only now being realized. Some experts believe that cows can be net carbon negative, although this topic is cause for debate.

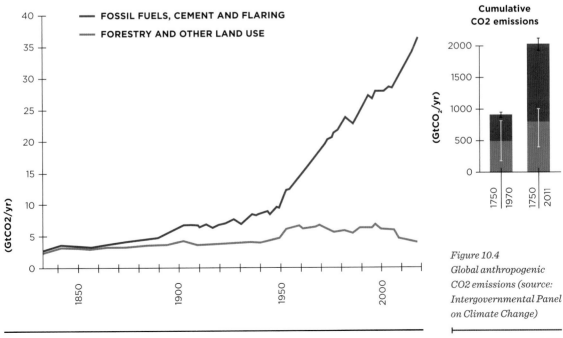

Figure 10.4
Global anthropogenic
CO2 emissions (source:
Intergovernmental Panel
on Climate Change)

If we look at the last 170 years or so, we see that the relative contribution to global greenhouse gas emissions from land usage, such as agriculture, has dramatically fallen compared to the use of things like fossil fuels. (Refer to Figure 10.4.) To shift the majority of the blame to ruminant animals, which have existed on the planet in far higher numbers than today, is misleading and inappropriate. Methane data included in these stats are in the form of CO_2 greenhouse gas equivalents. I also want to note that methane is considered a more "potent" greenhouse gas than CO_2, but it stays in the atmosphere for only a few years, whereas CO_2 hangs around for thousands of years. You also should realize that methane emissions from animals have been mostly stable over the last several decades, and the increase in methane in the atmosphere appears to be coming from other sources, such as a higher-than-predicted leakage from natural gas production.

Water usage is another issue that people cite when discussing the environmental concerns related to meat. The calculations of water use needed for livestock vary wildly depending on one's dietary political beliefs. Organizations such as PETA (People for the Ethical Treatment of Animals) cite extraordinary numbers—such as that it requires 2,400 gallons to make one pound of meat—typically reference green water, which is rainwater or snowfall in a field where an animal might eat. And while a small percentage of that rainwater ultimately contributes to growing grass or other foraged food for the animals, the ground absorbs most of it before it's returned to the atmosphere in the normal water cycle. Additionally, any water that cows drink doesn't just disappear from the earth forever. The cows urinate, defecate, and exhale water-filled breath; all that water returns to the atmosphere to once again fall as rain.

Figure 10.5 shows a more accurate breakdown of the numbers. You can see that, worldwide, rainwater (the green) represents approximately 94 percent of the water that goes into producing beef, and irrigated water (the blue) for drinking represents only about 3 percent. The remaining 3 percent is water needed to dilute and purify wastewater.

Meat's Water Footprint

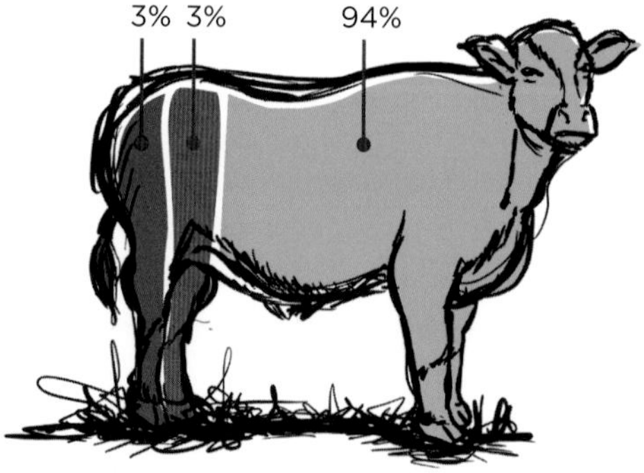

3% 3%   94%

DATA liter / kg

Green water

Blue water

Gray water

Total Water Footprint

15,415 liters

Figure 10.5
Water footprint
of worldwide cow
production (source:
UNESCO-IHE)

If we're genuinely concerned about the environmental impact of having animals, then we need to realize that there are more horses than dairy cows in the United States, and our pet population of cats and dogs exceeds 140 million animals, which directly compete with us for food resources when our diets include plants. The true environmentalist would also eliminate those animals from our environment. At least cows serve the purpose of feeding us, whereas the other animals are basically an environmental drain. I say this as a dog owner, and I have no intention of giving up my dogs. I'm only trying to demonstrate how biased the argument against meat has become.

You may hear some people say things such as, "Cows are destroying the Amazonian rain forest," or "To save the earth you need to give up the steak you're eating in Chicago." This type of statement is incredibly misleading. Firstly, that steak you eat in Chicago likely has zero effect on the Amazonian rain forest because only a tiny fraction of beef consumed in the United States comes from Brazil—far less than 1 percent. However, if you're concerned about this sort of thing, you could limit the effect by supporting the reinstitution of the Country of Origin Labeling laws that were in effect until a few years ago, so you'd know the exact country of origin of your beef. Most Brazilian beef goes to China, Hong Kong, and Russia. If you're looking to take up the fight to protect the rain forests, then go vegan in one of those countries.

CONTRIBUTORS TO DEFORESTATION

Cattle farming isn't the only cause of deforestation of the world's forests. Brazil produces about 120 million tons of soybeans and exports about 80 million tons of that to China, where much of it is turned into soybean oil for humans, and the waste products (in the form of soy meal) become feed for pigs. Another issue, not surprisingly, is wood production. And palm oil production is the leading cause of deforestation in Asia.

According to recent satellite imaging studies, forest cover in the United States and much of the rest of the world has increased in recent years. Certainly, no one condones further destruction of the rain forest, but not eating a steak in the United States, or in many other countries, has no effect on the rain forests in Brazil.

Before I leave the topic of environmental issues, I want to take a minute to talk about how issues are framed. Currently, the discussion about food and environmental impact is isolated to food production, and, as I've pointed out, even that issue is far more nuanced than the vegan proponents would have you believe. I want to step outside of that narrow focus for a bit to talk about food and environmental impact from another point of view.

Suppose we consider what happens after our food is produced and how it affects our environment. For example, according to the USDA, the average American eats roughly 2,000 pounds of food per year. We know from numerous surveys that the average person on a carnivore diet consumes roughly 1.5 to 2 pounds of food per day. When we extrapolate that to annual numbers, it works out to about 640 pounds per year, or about 32 percent of what everyone else is eating. Now, think about the reduction in transportation costs because of the smaller quantity of food consumed. If we also take into account that roughly 40 percent of the food we produce ends up in landfills—with the majority of it being fruits, vegetables, and baked goods—we also see significant environmental savings because we won't be wasting those things as we pursue a carnivore diet.

How much glass, plastic, cardboard, and metal goes into the packaging used for most of the food we buy? How much fossil fuel is used to produce that packaging? My household food-related trash is tiny compared to the amount of trash I used to produce when I was an omnivore.

Most carnivore dieters eat about twice per day. The average person consumes up to five or six meals and snacks per day. How much savings do we realize for electricity and gas needed to prepare two meals rather than six? What about the fact that much of the produce we eat is shipped from all over the world, but most of the meat we consume is domestically produced?

A carnivore's kitchen requires very little in the way of consumer goods. I typically use a cast-iron pan, a grill, a knife, a fork, and a plate. Compare that to the dozens of gadgets and cooking supplies most people use, and the carnivore diet wins here as well!

The U.S. healthcare system produces 10 percent of our greenhouse gas emissions. As I mention earlier in this chapter, U.S. cattle production is responsible for only about 2 percent of emissions, so there's another way in which the carnivore diet provides environmental savings. Alleviating certain health conditions places less burden on our healthcare system.

So my point with all these facts is this: When we're examining something as complex as our food system and the environment, let's take a broad view of the carnivore diet and not limit the discussion to the vegan proponents' favorite talking points.

Animal Population and Welfare

What if we could somehow set free all the animals that we now raise? What would happen to the 1.5 billion or so cows? Would they magically stop making methane? Would their populations migrate into urban or suburban areas? Cattle are fairly dangerous animals that can easily trample a human, and millions of them roaming around in populated areas would result in the loss of many human lives and countless injuries. What would happen to the millions of workers who depend on the animal agriculture industry for their livelihoods? What about the countless people whose health would decline without high-quality animal protein? Would we legalize the hunting of feral cows? How would those animals live and die? There are many issues to consider when you're discussing the ethics of raising animals to be used as food.

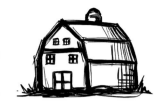

Vegans claim that we could feed more people on a plant-based diet. Although that is true from a purely caloric standpoint, we would see high percentages of the population develop severe nutritional deficiencies. Cattle have a more intense draw on resources, but they also provide an unmatched level of nutrition that plant food can't get close to. In particular, essential amino acids such as lysine would be difficult to obtain in sufficient quantities from a worldwide plant-based diet.

The answer is not to throw the baby out with the bathwater but to refine and improve the system. Farmers work constantly to address issues with the way they raise our food. During the last fifty years or so in the United States, farmers have tremendously reduced greenhouse gas emissions, land usage, water usage, and feed usage, and the efforts continue. Livestock is vital to human nutrition directly, but we also need them for plant agriculture. Animals play an essential role in soil replenishment, which benefits plant agriculture, and provide far more benefit than we typically recognize. It's impossible to have an agricultural system that doesn't include animals.

Let's talk about the issue of animal welfare, which is incredibly important. I've had the privilege of speaking with many cattle ranchers when I've visited ranches and feedlots. Most people don't get that opportunity, so when they're exposed to propaganda against animal agriculture, they don't have any firsthand experience to compare it to. To be clear, a minority of people in the industry don't do a good job, and it is these people whom the propaganda folks use as examples. Most of the people who grow up with, spend their lives learning about, and make a living from animals are incredibly caring, and they do everything in their power to keep the animals in their charge safe and healthy. In no way whatsoever does it benefit a rancher, or even a feedlot owner, to have a sick, stressed out, or otherwise compromised animal. Furthermore, in the United States and many other countries, there are numerous regulations to ensure animal welfare, and the consequences of not complying with those regulations are significant.

Animal rights advocates often point out that newborn animals frequently are removed from direct proximity to their mothers shortly after birth. The reason for their removal is not some nefarious purpose but to protect the infant from being accidentally killed by its mother or to prevent infection or malnutrition. Accidental deaths of newborn animals are

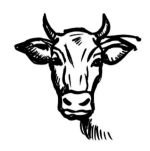

not uncommon; some animals accidentally kill up to 90 percent of their litters. However, this type of detail is not something the PETA zealots will tell you.

Despite what countless family films about anthropomorphic farm animals might have us believe, the animals we eat are neither our pets nor our friends. Ultimately, they are essential food for our survival and health. Feeding the mass of humanity is a task of enormous magnitude, and a lot of animals are unquestionably a key component of completing that task. Some ranchers will tell you how they sometimes bring sick calves into their homes or how they're in the field seven days a week in the rain or snow to take care of their animals. If you talk to some pen riders, who oversee cattle housed in feed yards, they will explain that they meticulously look at every single animal every single day to ensure that they are doing well and remaining healthy. The people who raise the animals we eat for food take their jobs seriously.

Yes, we have to slaughter these animals to obtain the various products we use from their flesh, but animals in the wild suffer far more than animals on ranches or feedlots. For example, animals raised on ranches or feedlots experience a quick, humane death. In the wild, a significant percentage of ruminant animals die long before adulthood, often as hungry predators eviscerate them while they're still alive. Most full-grown animals die the same way and spend every day of their lives trying to avoid that fate. Animals who don't die by predation suffer from terminal injuries or diseases, or often they starve to death.

The idea that cows are locked in pens with no place to turn around as they're force-fed grains as soon as they're born is an absolute joke. By regulation, cattle have far more room in the feed yard than they ever will use. The reason they cluster together is that they are herd animals, and it's their instinct to huddle up as protection against predators. Also, be aware that the vast majority of cattle spend most of their lives in the pasture. In fact, of the 90 million or so cattle in the United States, only around 14 million of them will be in a feed yard at any one time because they spend most of their time out munching grass, shrubs, and other stuff we humans have no nutritional use for. Food that's inedible to humans comprises approximately 86 percent of a cow's lifetime diet; cattle also often eat much of the by-products from the production of our food. Those by-products would otherwise go to landfills and contribute greatly to global pollution.

Temple Grandin, whom I met several years ago at a lecture on autism (my eldest son has autism spectrum disorder), has been a huge driving force within the United States for the humane treatment of animals as they are processed for slaughter. The Glass Walls Project from the American Meat Institute provides a real-world, no-holds-barred look into the way animals are processed from day to day. You can find the AMI's videos, which are hosted by Dr. Grandin, on YouTube, and I encourage you to view these videos rather than relying on vegan propaganda films that often show third-world practices that no one in the United States (or almost any other developed country) supports.

Countering Vegans' Arguments

I want to address some of the statements from vegans in defense of the claim that humans are herbivores. (And I'll go on the record as saying that I think these statements are idiotic.) For a second, I'll ignore the fact that humans have been eating meat for as long as humans have existed—probably at least as long as 3 million years. Heck, even chimpanzees aggressively eat meat when they can get it. In Africa, red colobus monkeys are at risk for endangerment because chimpanzees hunt them. If humans were truly herbivores, why did we not depart from eating animals 10,000 or so years ago when agriculture began to take off?

I enjoy it when someone confronts me and states that if humans were meant to eat meat, then we should chase down our prey, kill it with our claws and teeth, and then eat it raw and whole. This statement is just ridiculous. If we want to dismiss 3 million years of evolution during which we developed tools, advanced hunting techniques, and the capacity to cook, then perhaps the argument might have a tiny amount of merit. This idea also discounts the fact that even today many people still eat and enjoy raw meats without any problems. We could flip the question around and ask how people would fare if they had to open coconuts with their teeth or eat unprocessed beans or nuts. Perhaps vegan proponents could explain how they would survive year-round eating only local fruits in places like Canada without having any tools or other ways to preserve food.

This next argument is related to the first: Humans can't eat meat because we don't have sharp claws or pointy teeth. The biggest carnivorous animal on the planet (the blue whale) has no teeth and certainly does not have claws. Countless nonhuman animals have learned to use tools to access food. Crows, octopuses, chimpanzees, elephants, sea otters, dolphins, gorillas, orangutans, rodents, and macaques have been observed using tools. Humans' jaw structure changed as we developed the capacity to use tools and speak. We no longer require jaws powerful enough to tear raw flesh from bone, although it is still quite easy to find humans who do just that.

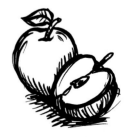

Another argument I often hear is that we must be herbivores because humans' stomach acid isn't very acidic. I'm not sure that the people who make up this stuff even pretend to research their claims. The stomach acid of a healthy human has been shown to have a pH of 1.1 to 1.5, which makes our stomachs among the most acidic environments in the entire animal kingdom. Numerous studies have confirmed this range, and one can easily find this detail in a basic gastrointestinal physiology textbook.

Vegans will tell you that veganism will absolve you of any guilt associated with animal death as it pertains to acquiring food. However, a study published in *Journal of Agriculture and Environmental Ethics* examined incidental death of field animals that occurred as a result of growing and harvesting crops in the United States, and the estimate is that 7.3 billion animals die annually. Although it would be impossible to get an exact count, we can safely say it's far more than the approximately 40 million cows that are sacrificed each year to feed us, and the quantity is close to the number of chickens that die each year. It's safe to say that many millions of animals' lives are lost regardless of your diet (unless you are a breatharian, which is a whole new level of crazy). Who determines that a cow's life is more important than that of a rabbit, mouse, or turkey?

Here are some other things I wonder: Does the destruction of an entire ecosystem to support growing crops of strawberries lend itself to better sleep at night than eating a steak? The United States imports 50 percent of all fruit consumed. Are people who are concerned about the environmental cost or potential human exploitation in other countries worried about that? Does the fact that huge amounts of those same fruits end up as waste bother anyone?

If you decide to go vegan, and it is perfectly within your right to do so, don't pretend your choice is about health. At best a vegan diet is no better than any other non-SAD diet, and at worst it's a recipe for health disaster. Also, don't pretend that the choice is about saving the environment because, in all honesty, veganism has a relatively minuscule effect. You can say it will prevent the humane dispatch of a small number of select animal species. What would become of those animals if we didn't eat them is unclear, but likely many would actually have a shorter, more painful existence, and almost certainly they would have much more traumatic and painful deaths.

If the purpose of veganism is to minimize harm to animals and to benefit the environment, then, to be true to that purpose, one needs to become a strict meat-based eater who eats only animals raised in a regenerative fashion as they are in places like Joel Salatin's Polyface Farm. This style of food production eliminates pesticides and biodiversity-destroying mono-cropping, causes the fewest animal deaths, and has a net positive effect on the soil and general ecosystem. Vegans should direct their efforts into supporting regenerative agriculture rather than angrily protesting, because that type of farming represents a clear step in the right direction; it will lead to a better environment and happier, healthier human animals.

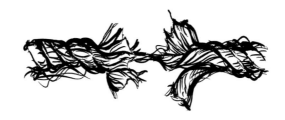

CHAPTER ELEVEN

LOOSE ENDS AND ODD BITS

Now that I've covered the major topics, only a few loose ends and odd bits remain for me to tell you about the carnivore diet. In this chapter, I cover some of the practical aspects of transitioning to a meat-based lifestyle.

Affordability of the Carnivore Diet

One of the most common questions people ask me is, "How can you afford to go on a meat-based diet?" Typically, high-quality protein is the most expensive part of a meal, and for a good reason. Animal-sourced protein is superior in amino acid completeness, bioavailability, and overall nutrition. Beef is an incredible-tasting superfood, and organ meats, if you enjoy them, are even higher in nutrition.

If cost is a concern—which it is for most people, including me—it pays to get smart about your purchases. If you prefer to eat organic or grass-finished beef, you feel it's of additional benefit, and you can afford the luxury, then, by all means, buy it. If you're not in the position to take on the extra expense, or you don't think the taste is worth the price, then buy the grain-fed beef that's widely available at supermarkets. There's nothing wrong with the grain-fed beef, and you shouldn't feel guilty or pressured by others not to buy it.

Finding affordable meat can require some planning, but the work will be worth the reward. Buying in bulk and freezing is an effective strategy. I often buy 40 or 50 pounds at a time from a supermarket when the price is right. Websites such as MyGroceryDeals.com make finding great sales easy. At these types of sites, you type *steak* in the Search field and your ZIP Code in the Near This Location field to find the best prices in your area. Meat is often heavily discounted just before major holidays, so that's a good time to stock up. Another option is to work with a local rancher or to contract directly with a local processor to get a half or quarter cow.

Different cuts of meat lend themselves to different cooking techniques. Some of the leaner cuts can be made very tender with various slow-cooking and low-temperature methods. Ground beef is often inexpensive and is a delicious option. Organ meats tend to be very cost friendly, and they probably provide more nutrition per dollar than any other food.

Get to know your local butcher, and you likely can get some great deals. Some butchers will throw in stuff—like trimmed fats, organs, and bones, which you can use to make broth or to cook with—for free.

Another cost-effective way to supplement your diet is to include eggs in your meals. Eggs often are inexpensively priced.

Cooking Methods

The scope of this book doesn't allow for a course in cooking, but I have some general comments. Cooking is an essential skill, and it's particularly critical to learn how to cook a decent steak properly. There's much debate about the best cooking method for steak, but I advise you to try out several to find the one that suits you best.

Grilling meat over a flame is hundreds of thousands of years old, and it still works pretty darn well. Charcoal, wood pellets, and gas are some of the fuel options. Different fire sources impart different flavors to the meat, and this is especially true with different types of wood. It's not uncommon for people to determine which fuel source is their favorite for the flavor they like best.

Eating grilled meat does not cause cancer, and the evidence to suggest that it might is not credible. Therefore, cooking the meat so it has a slight char is unlikely to cause any health problems. If you can show me the study that demonstrates that actual humans with a functioning liver eating only meat with a slight char on it develop cancer, I'll change my tune on this. If you burn the meat to a crisp, perhaps it's a problem, but burnt meat is no longer edible, of course, and shame on you for overcooking it.

After you've grilled a few dozen steaks, you'll get pretty good at sizing up the situation. You'll instinctively know when to turn the steak and how long to cook it to get it to your preferred doneness. Early on, be prepared to stay close by at all times and watch things carefully. The thickness of the cut, the type of steak, and the fat content are all going to affect your cooking strategy.

Searing a steak in a pan is another common preparation technique. If you like your steaks rare, this method can be the quickest way to get the job done. You don't even need to add cooking fat because you can use rendered fat from the steak itself. I often heat the pan, preferably cast iron, until it's very hot; then I touch the fatty edge of the steak to the pan to form a shallow layer of hot cooking fat. After that, I sear the steak. Alternatively, you can use ghee or butter, or you can use animal fats like tallow, lard, or bacon grease. To bring your game up a notch, learn how to reverse sear the steak, which involves slowly cooking the steak at a relatively low temperature until the internal temperature reaches your desired doneness. Then you place the steak in a hot pan to sear both sides quickly and achieve the perfect finish. Adding spices and herbs, if you tolerate them, can impart a nice flavor to the meat with any of these cooking techniques.

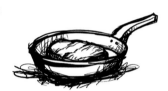

Sous vide, which is French for *under vacuum*, is another neat technique that many people swear by for getting the perfect steak. It involves placing the steak in a plastic bag and putting it in a precisely controlled water bath for a relatively long time, as long as forty-eight hours. When you take the steak out of the bath, you sear it in a pan or with a blow torch. The result is an incredibly tender and perfectly flavored cut of meat. Wow, my mouth is watering just thinking about it!

Some people favor broiling as a cooking method. In my experience, though, the outcome isn't as good as the previous options.

You can try various slow cooking techniques for leaner cuts and roasts; these methods can be a great way to prepare a large amount of meat to have on hand. Multicookers, like the Instant Pot, and other pressure-cooking devices can significantly shorten cooking times for tougher cuts of meat while still producing results that are similar to more traditional slow cooker methods. The good old-fashioned oven is another good tool for preparing a roast.

A relatively newcomer to the food gadget world is the Air Fryer. I've cooked steaks with it several times, and I can say it's a very good option for convenience and ease of use.

Traveling on the Carnivore Diet

Let's talk a little about being on the road as a carnivore. In the United States, it's pretty unusual not to find a town that, at the very least, has a restaurant that sells hamburgers. Yes, fast food hamburger restaurants, which have a heck of a lot of garbage on the menu, do have one thing that is actually a health food—beef! Despite what you might have heard, the majority of fast food restaurants use 100 percent ground beef. The restaurants typically cook the burgers without any added oils, and they usually don't contain any fillers, although some restaurants may add spices that can be problematic for some people.

When I go to a fast food restaurant, the first thing I do is ask if they sell individual burger patties. The answer is almost always yes. Then I inquire about the price, which typically is about $1.50 or so for a quarter pound of beef (depending on the geographic location). At that point, I drop the bombshell and order eight to twelve patties. Sometimes I add a few strips of bacon and occasionally cheese, but most of the time I get only the burgers. This is a wonderfully cheap way to get some delicious, nutrient-dense, freshly cooked food relatively inexpensively. In my opinion, we likely could solve our obesity crisis and address many chronic disease issues if people would go to these fast food places and eat nothing but fresh beef. I'm sure some heads are ready to explode after reading the preceding statement, but that's the way it is. The very fast food institutions that have largely contributed to the chronic disease epidemic can also go a long way to helping with the cure! (I look forward to receiving all kinds of hate mail.)

Prepared steaks that have been cut up can be an excellent source of road food; I often take them with me. I cook them, cut them, sprinkle them with a little salt, and put them in a plastic bag or another container so I can eat them while I'm traveling. Beef jerky, pemmican, and biltong are all decent travel foods that you can purchase; even better, you can make them at home, so you have greater control over the ingredients. You can take boiled eggs, bacon, and even small amounts of cheese on the road. Sausages and other processed meat can be a nice snack, but I suggest you carefully look at the ingredients and avoid varieties with soy, gluten, heavy sugars, and other undesirable ingredients. Certainly, you shouldn't make these types of meats the center of your diet, but they'll do for an occasional snack or travel food.

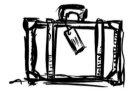

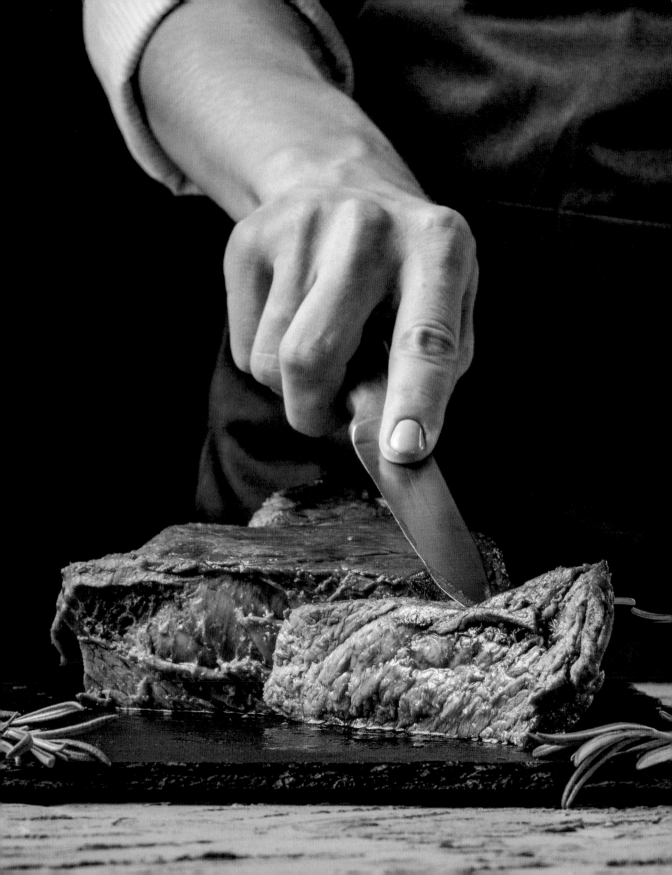

Resources

Because the carnivore diet has an ever-growing fan base, there are quite a few online resources that you may find useful as you transition to the diet. Here are some of my favorites:

- **Cholesterol Code** (*cholesterolcode.com*): This website run by Dave Feldman talks about all things cholesterol, including how to dramatically change the levels of it in your body.

- **Diagnosis: Diet** (*diagnosisdiet.com*): Dr. Georgia Ede provides lots of great info on problems with plants and why the evidence that red meat causes cancer is weak.

- **Dr. Malcolm Kendrick** (*drmalcomkendrick.org*): Dr. Malcolm Kendrick is a physician from Scotland who writes and speaks about heart disease and other health issues.

- **The Fat Emperor** (*thefatemperor.com*): This is the online home for Ivor Cummins, who provides excellent information about cholesterol, insulin, and disease risk.

- **Just Eat Meat** (*justmeat.co*): This website has an amazing compendium of resources for information about the carnivore diet. The site includes an extensive list of articles and books on the subject; a compilation of social media accounts; a wiki of pages related to the diet; and information about the various world cultures that have thrived on meat-based diets.

- **The Ketogenic Diet for Health** (*ketotic.org*): Amber O'Hearn, who has been a carnivore since 2009, and Zooko run this blog filled with brilliant posts about the carnivore and ketogenic diets.

- **Meat Heals** (*meatheals.com*): This site has an ever-growing collection of testimonials from people who've experienced health transformations after they've adopted a meat-based diet.

- **Principia Carnivora** (*www.facebook.com/groups/PrincipiaCarnivora/*): This is the largest private carnivore Facebook group, with more than 20,000 members.

- **Protein Power** (*proteinpower.com*): This website offers great information from long-time low-carb pioneers Drs. Michael and Mary Dan Eades.

- **Tuit Nutrition** (*tuitnutrition.com*): Author Amy Berger has a master's degree in human nutrition. On her website, she provides great overall nutrition advice in a very enjoyable writing style.

- **World Carnivore Tribe** (*www.facebook.com/groups/worldcarnivoretribe/*): This is my public Facebook group. The more than 28,000 members share their knowledge, experience, and data to support one another in the quest for better health through a carnivore diet.

- **Zeroing in on Health** (*www.facebook.com/groups/zioh2/*): This is another well-established public Facebook group. Eleven-year carnivore veteran Charles Washington administers the site.

Wrapping Up

No matter how you end up implementing your carnivore diet, I think the biggest takeaway is that meat is a crucial part of human nutrition. For many, meat is completely sufficient and is incredibly health-giving. Others can use the diet as a high-powered tool to figure out food intolerances or to combat health challenges. Athletes may find that going carnivore improves their performance, body composition, and recovery dramatically. Many may choose to use it cyclically. Others may choose to remain "mostly carnivorous" and thrive that way.

I can promise you that going carnivore will neither enable you to save the broccoli of the world from maltreatment nor get you a free pass into heaven. You will be no more morally superior than anyone else, and your vibration frequencies or karmic balance will not be improved. But I hope you will come to have a better relationship with nutrition and learn a little bit more about your physiology.

I thank you for purchasing and reading this book, and I hope you'll share some of this information with those you feel might benefit from it. The carnivore diet is an evolving topic in the health and nutrition field, and I expect to see a great deal more knowledge becoming available shortly. Several brilliant people—such as Amber O'Hearn, Dr. Paul Saladino, and Dr. Ted Naiman—will soon be adding to the discussion. I look forward to seeing the work of those people and hope those of you who have supported me will also lend other carnivore diet advocates your support. It will take a huge effort from everyone at the grassroots level to turn this out-of-control train around and take back our health and our happiness.

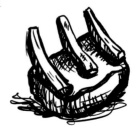

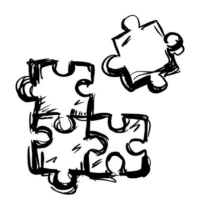

EPILOGUE

Ultimately, you should eat however you choose, and I hope you'll factor your health into that equation. Over the coming years, I think we're going to witness a battle for how we're allowed to eat, and the results are going to affect us for generations. Some people are expressing a great desire for us to move away from meat. Most people won't want to, and thus these groups are employing strategies to coax us in that direction.

At first, we'll be asked nicely to cut back on our meat consumption. Certain powers will use claims about health risks, environmental damage, and concern for humane treatment of animals to convince us to comply. As I've pointed out, you can't boil nutrition down to simple black-and-white "do this, not that" explanations; people who do that are ignoring a tremendous amount of context. In 1977, then Senator George McGovern announced that he didn't have the luxury to wait on science; the result of his impatience is that we were saddled with the disastrous U.S. Food Guidelines.

Today we're in a similar situation, and the same sort of thing is happening. We're being told to give up eating the food that our species relied on because we're told that the sacrifice will save the planet. The science on this is far from final, and there are many dissenting voices. There are myriad ways in which we can proceed, and the so-called easy solution of getting rid of the cows has a frighteningly high number of potentially disastrous results. That solution might help in the short term, but short-term solutions rarely work for the long haul. Just as in the medical field, where high-tech bandages are routinely applied to limit symptoms, the removal of animal agriculture does not address the true issues at the heart of our food systems.

Grazing animals in the grasslands have been on the earth for 10 million years; they are not the problem. We have seen significant reductions in our grasslands, and we've watched large swathes of lands turn to desert. These issues can be reversed through well-managed pasturing of ruminant animals. We should be maximizing every single scrap of pastureland and getting as many cows on it as possible. Lab-grown meat and its heavy reliance on monocropped agriculture is not going to be a long-term solution; it'll send us further down the path of turning the planet into a dust bowl. Investors see a multibillion-dollar opportunity in selling more processed food disguised as "meat alternatives," and they're pushing hard to convince us that we need these products. The result will be nonstop media campaigns and reports from paid-for science. The people behind this movement are preying on our weakness and our lack of capacity for individual thought.

If we don't comply willingly, the government will apply legislative pressures. Draconian consumer taxes, tariffs, trade policies, and other restrictions will take place. As I said earlier, I've heard many of my fellow carnivores say, "They'll have to pry the rib-eye from my cold, dead hands." That's a nice sentiment, but unfortunately the rib-eye will never make it into your hands in the first place. It will be so darn expensive that many people will opt to make do with soybean slop or fake lab Franken-Meat. For those of you who say you'll take up hunting, know that the U.S. deer population is only about 30 million animals. If a large increase in the number of hunters were to occur, those animals would be gone quickly.

As long as people remain addicted to sugar and other junk food, nothing will change. We'll continue to accept a pathetic existence and call it a normal consequence of aging. You'll be sold supplements to counteract the damaging effects of drugs you take to treat the conditions that are caused by the garbage diet you eat. You'll be fed the equivalent of human pet food, and you'll like it. The manufacturers will engineer it to be tasty—that's for sure—but there won't be any nutritional value in it. I don't know about you guys, but the thought of this just pisses me off!

What can you do if you don't want to see a future in which processed food is our mainstay? If you don't want to be placated by "peasant food" or make do with heaps of cheap grain, sugar, and highly processed oils and only a few scraps of meat that will keep you from dying right away, then you need to act today. It may already be too late, but I'm not going down without a fight, and I hope you won't either.

On December 16, 1773, an angry mob of protesters dumped 342 chests of tea into the Boston harbor to demonstrate their displeasure with what they felt were unfair and inappropriate tax policies. This act contributed to the start of the American Revolutionary war. Today our subjugation is not being carried out by a foreign army but rather by an insidious system of low-quality foods and mindless entertainment. Will we sit passively by as our bodies decay? I'm not interested in that path.

Make no mistake; in the battle for our food future, every weapon available will be used to force you to comply. I don't see how we can sit idly by and wait to be told what to do and what to eat. When I first started this journey of recovering my health, I had no idea that I would have to resort to activism to protect my capacity to take care of my body. Can a population of people come together, organize, and direct their own future, or will greed, corporate interests, and apathy prevail? If you're reading this and you want to help, regardless of whether you follow this diet, get involved. Use social media, contact your local politicians, let the processed food companies know that you don't want their crappy offerings anymore, teach your children about nutrition, and challenge what you're being told. The carnivore diet is ultimately about much more than just eating meat. It's about regaining one's life and one's freedom!

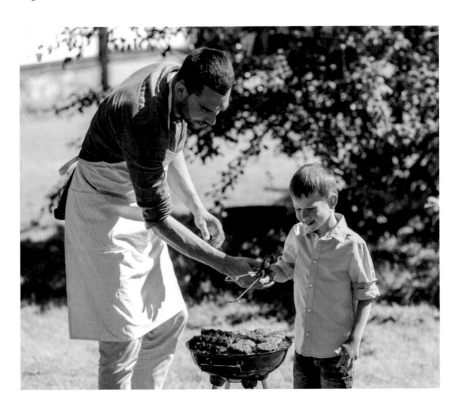

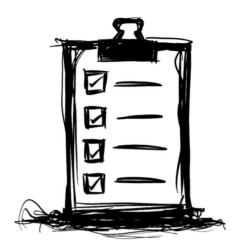

CARNIVORE
CHEAT SHEET

In this handy reference guide, I've provided some information to help you plan and shop for your carnivore meals. Although you could go to the grocery to load up on lots of rib-eye steaks, ground beef, and bacon, you may want to mix it up from time to time by incorporating other meats. In this appendix, I share nutritional information about various meat and dairy products, diagrams of the cuts of meat on various livestock, cooking temperatures for beef, and an explanation of the USDA's grading system for beef.

First, though, here are a few carnivore-friendly websites that you may want to check out:

- **ButcherBox** (*butcherbox.com*)
- **Cabriejo Ranch** (*cabriejoranch.com*)
- **Certified Piedmontese** (*piedmontese.com*)
- **Colorado Craft Beef** (*coloradocraftbeef.com*)
- **Eatwild** (*eatwild.com/*)
- **Epic Provisions** (*epicprovisions.com*)
- **Mountain Primal Beef Co.** (*mountainprimal.com*)
- **Polyface Farms** (*polyfacefarms.com/food-sales/*)
- **The Provision House** (*theprovisionhouse.com*)
- **Savory** (*savory.global*)
- **Thousand Hills** (*thousandhillslifetimegrazed.com*)
- **U.S. Wellness Meats** (*grasslandbeef.com*)
- **White Oak Pastures** (*whiteoakpastures.com*)

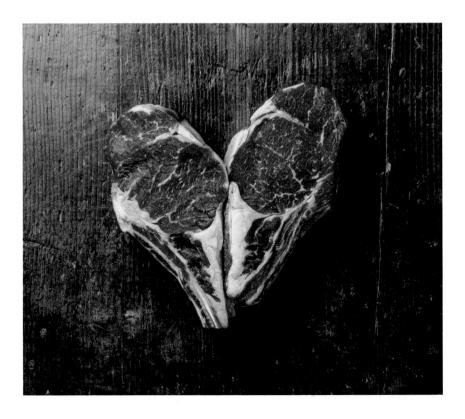

Nutritional Information

The following table lists nutritional information for various foods that you may include in your carnivore diet.

BEEF (4 OUNCES)	Calories	Fat	Protein	Carbs	Fiber	P/E ratio	Nutrients
Tenderloin steak	115	3.0	22.2	0.0	0.0	7.40	
Testicles	154	3.4	29.7	1.14	0	6.54	Zinc, iron, phosphorus, and potassium
Heart	187	5.4	32.2	0.2	0.0	5.96	B12, potassium, selenium, collagen
Kidney	179	5.3	31.0	0.0	0.0	5.85	Omega-3, B12, iron
Shank cross cut	215	6.7	38.7	0.0	0.0	5.80	
Sirloin tip side steak	190	6.0	34.0	0.0	0.0	5.67	
Liver	216	6.0	33.0	5.8	0.0	5.50	Almost everything, especially vitamins A, C, and D, folate, and minerals like magnesium, selenium, potassium, and zinc
Sirloin tip center roast	190	7.0	31.0	0.0	0.0	4.43	
Sirloin tip center steak	190	7.0	31.0	0.0	0.0	4.43	
Shoulder pot roast	185	7.0	30.7	0.0	0.0	4.38	
Flank steak	200	8.0	32.0	0.0	0.0	4.00	
Round tip steak	150	6.0	23.5	0.0	0.0	3.92	
Shoulder petite tender	150	7.0	22.0	0.0	0.0	3.14	
Shoulder petite tender medallions	150	7.0	22.0	0.0	0.0	3.14	
Tenderloin roast	180	8.0	25.0	0.0	0.0	3.13	
Shoulder center ranch steak	152	8.0	24.0	0.0	0.0	3.00	
Tripe (intestines)	107	4.6	13.3	2.3	0.0	2.89	Selenium, B12, and zinc
Top round steak	180	9.0	25.0	0.0	0.0	2.78	
Eye of round steak	182	9.0	25.0	0.0	0.0	2.78	
Chuck steak, boneless	160	8.0	22.0	0.0	0.0	2.75	
Eye of round roast	253	13.4	32.0	0.0	0.0	2.39	
Tri-tip steak	200	11.0	23.0	0.0	0.0	2.09	
Shoulder steak	204	12.0	24.0	0.0	0.0	2.00	

continues on next page

BEEF (4 OUNCES)	Calories	Fat	Protein	Carbs	Fiber	P/E ratio	Nutrients
Chuck pot roast, 7-bone	240	14.0	28.0	0.0	0.0	2.00	
Chuck pot roast, boneless	240	14.0	28.0	0.0	0.0	2.00	
Brisket, flat cut	245	14.7	28.0	0.0	0.0	1.91	
Round tip roast	199	12.0	22.9	0.0	0.0	1.91	
Shoulder top blade steak	204	13.0	22.0	0.0	0.0	1.69	
Shoulder top blade flat iron steak	204	13.0	22.0	0.0	0.0	1.69	
Bottom round roast	220	14.0	23.0	0.0	0.0	1.64	
Bottom round steak	220	14.0	23.0	0.0	0.0	1.64	
Skirt steak	255	16.5	27.0	0.0	0.0	1.64	
Top sirloin steak	240	16.0	22.0	0.0	0.0	1.38	
T-bone	170	12.2	15.8	0.0	0.0	1.30	
Chuck eye steak	250	18.0	21.0	0.0	0.0	1.17	
Brains	171	11.9	13.2	1.7	0.0	1.11	Cholesterol, omega-3, selenium, copper, and B5
Top loin steak, bone-in	270	20.0	21.0	0.0	0.0	1.05	
Top loin steak, boneless	270	20.0	21.0	0.0	0.0	1.05	
Rib roast	373	28.0	27.0	0.0	0.0	0.96	
Porterhouse	280	22.0	21.0	0.0	0.0	0.95	
Sweetbreads	362	28.3	25.0	0.0	0.0	0.88	Vitamins C and K, omega-3, selenium, phosphorus, and zinc
Tongue	322	25.3	22.0	0.0	0.0	0.87	Vitamins D and B, choline, iron, and zinc
Rib-eye steak	310	25.0	20.0	0.0	0.0	0.80	
Back ribs	310	26.0	19.0	0.0	0.0	0.73	
Tri-tip roast	340	29.0	18.0	0.0	0.0	0.62	
Short ribs, boneless	440	41.0	16.0	0.0	0.0	0.39	

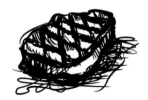

FISH AND SEAFOOD (4 OUNCES)	Calories	Fat	Protein	Carbs	Fiber	P/E ratio	Nutrients
Shrimp	112	0.32	27.2	0.23	0	49.45	
Langostino	93	0.67	21.3	0	0	31.79	
Tuna (canned)	149	1.06	32.91	0	0	31.05	
Northern pike	128	1.0	28.0	0	0	28.00	
Cod	113	1.0	26.0	0	0	26.00	
Orange roughy	119	1.0	25.7	0	0	25.70	
Crab	94	0.84	20.28	0	0	24.14	
Tuna (yellowfin)	150	1.5	34.0	0	0	22.67	
Lobster	101	1.0	22.0	0	0	22.00	
Crappie	132	1.34	28.2	0	0	21.04	
Bluegill	133	1.34	28.2	0	0	21.04	
Perch	132	1.34	28.2	0	0	21.04	
Mahi mahi	100	1.0	21.0	0	0	21.00	
Grouper	134	1.5	28.2	0	0	18.80	
Crayfish (crawfish)	93	1.4	19.0	0	0	13.57	
Barramundi	110	2.0	23.0	0	0	11.50	
Tilapia	145	3.0	29.7	0	0	9.90	
Monkfish	110	2.2	21.1	0	0	9.59	
Sea bass	135	3.0	27.0	0	0	9.00	
Halibut	155	3.5	30.7	0	0	8.77	
Salmon roe (ikura)	185	4.0	34.3	0	0	8.58	
Catfish	119	3.2	20.9	0	0	6.53	
Flounder	97.5	2.7	17.3	0	0	6.41	
Turbot	138	4.3	23.3	0	0	5.42	
Octopus	186	2.4	33.8	5	0	4.57	
Squid	119	1.8	20.3	4	0	3.50	
Salmon	206	9.0	31.0	0	0	3.44	
Scallops	126	1.0	23.0	6	0	3.29	
Trout	190	8.6	28.0	0	0	3.26	
Swordfish	195	9.0	26.6	0	0	2.96	
Walleye	156	7.5	22.0	0	0	2.93	
Arctic char	208	10.0	29.0	0	0	2.90	
Cockle	90	0.8	15.3	5.3	0	2.51	
Fish livers	118	5.0	12.5	5.8	0.0	2.50	Almost everything, especially vitamins A, C, and D, folate, and minerals like magnesium, selenium, potassium, and zinc

continues on next page

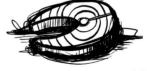

FISH AND SEAFOOD (4 OUNCES)	Calories	Fat	Protein	Carbs	Fiber	P/E ratio	Nutrients
Sardines	139	7.5	18.0	0	0	2.40	
Mussels	195	5.0	27.0	8.38	0	2.02	
Clams	161	6.7	27.5	6.7	0	2.05	
Sea urchin	137	5.6	18.3	3.9	0	1.93	
Anchovies	256	15.9	28.0	0	0	1.76	
Eel	267	17.0	26.8	0	0	1.58	
Mackerel	290	20.3	27.0	0	0	1.33	
Oysters	92	2.6	10.7	5.6	0	1.30	
Herring	283.5	20.2	23.8	0	0	1.18	
Caviar	299	20.3	27.9	4.54	0	1.12	
Escargot	21.6	0.2	1.3	3.5	3.2	0.35	

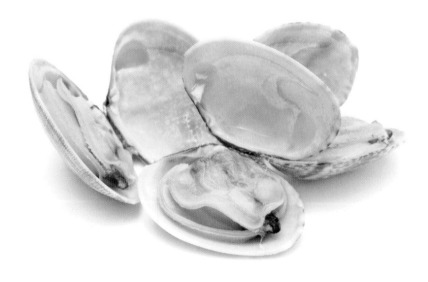

PORK (4 OUNCES)	Calories	Fat	Protein	Carbs	Fiber	P/E ratio	Nutrients
Tenderloin	158	4.0	30.0	0	0	7.50	
Liver	187	5.0	29.5	4.3	0.0	5.90	Almost everything, especially vitamins A, C, and D, folate, and minerals like magnesium, selenium, potassium, and zinc
Kidney	171	5.3	28.8	0.0	0.0	5.43	Omega-3, B12, and iron
Heart	168	5.7	26.8	0.5	0.0	4.70	B12, potassium, selenium, and collagen
Chop	241	12.0	33.0	0	0	2.75	
Rump	280	16.2	32.8	0	0	2.02	
Loin	265	15.5	30.8	0	0	1.99	
Middle ribs (country style)	245	16.0	25.0	0	0	1.56	
Leg ham	305	20.0	30.4	0	0	1.52	
Ears	188	12.3	18.0	0.2	0.0	1.46	Collagen, choline, vitamin D, and calcium
Tongue	307	21.0	27.3	0.0	0.0	1.30	Vitamins B and D, choline, iron, and zinc
Brains	156	11.0	14.0	0.0	0.0	1.27	Cholesterol, omega-3, selenium, copper, and vitamin B5
Butt	240	18.0	19.0	0	0	1.06	
Cracklings (pork rinds)	530	40.0	39.0	1.9	0.0	0.98	Collagen
Bacon	600	47.2	41.8	0	0	0.89	
Shoulder	285	23.0	19.0	0	0	0.83	
Hocks	285	24.0	17.0	0	0	0.71	
Loin back ribs (baby back ribs)	315	27.0	18.0	0	0	0.67	
Belly	588	60.0	10.4	0	0	0.17	

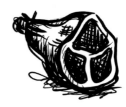

CHICKEN AND POULTRY (4 OUNCES)	Calories	Fat	Protein	Carbs	Fiber	P/E ratio	Nutrients
Chicken gizzards	175	3.0	34.5	0.0	0.0	11.50	Niacin, zinc, selenium, and iron
Chicken breast, skinless	138	4.0	25.0	0	0	6.25	
Chicken giblets (kidney)	178	5.1	30.8	0.0	0.0	6.04	Omega-3, B12, and iron
Chicken liver	189	7.4	27.7	1.0	0.0	3.74	Almost everything, especially vitamins A, C, and D, folate, and minerals like magnesium, selenium, potassium, and zinc
Chicken breast, skin-on	200	8.4	31.0	0	0	3.69	
Chicken heart	210	9.0	30.0	0.1	0.0	3.33	Vitamin B12, potassium, selenium, and collagen
Chicken leg, skinless	210	9.5	30.7	0	0	3.23	
Pheasant	200	10.5	25.7	0	0	2.45	
Chicken drums	178	9.9	22.0	0	0	2.22	
Turkey	175	9.9	21.0	0	0	2.12	
Chicken leg, skin-on	255	15.2	29.4	0	0	1.93	
Chicken thigh, skinless	165	10.0	19.0	0	0	1.90	
Duck	228	13.9	26.3	0	0	1.89	
Chicken thigh, skin-on	275	17.6	28.3	0	0	1.61	
Chicken wings	320	22.0	30.4	0	0	1.38	
Chicken feet	244	16.6	22.0	0.2	0.0	1.33	Collagen, riboflavin, calcium, and hyaluronic acid
Game hen	220	16.0	19.0	0	0	1.19	
Goose	340	24.9	28.5	0	0	1.14	
Chicken skin	514	46.0	23.0	0.0	0.0	0.50	Collagen, calcium, and oleic acid

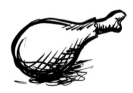

GOAT AND LAMB (4 OUNCES)	Calories	Fat	Protein	Carbs	Fiber	P/E ratio	Nutrients
Goat meat	162	3.4	30.7	0	0	9.03	
Goat ribs	162	3.4	30.7	0	0	9.03	
Goat oysters (testicles)	154	3.4	29.7	1.14	0	6.54	Zinc, iron, phosphorus, and potassium
Lamb oysters (testicles)	154	3.4	29.7	1.14	0	6.54	Zinc, iron, phosphorus, and potassium
Goat liver	217	5.9	33.0	5.8	0	2.82	Almost everything, especially vitamins A, C, and D, folate, and minerals like magnesium, selenium, potassium, and zinc
Lamb liver	250	10.0	34.7	2.87	0	2.70	Almost everything, especially vitamins A, C, and D, folate, and minerals like magnesium, selenium, potassium, and zinc
Lamb chops	313	22.7	25.5	0	0	1.12	
Lamb, ground	313	22.7	25.5	0	0	1.12	

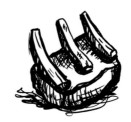

WILD GAME (4 OUNCES)	Calories	Fat	Protein	Carbs	Fiber	P/E ratio	Nutrients
Venison loin*	169.3	2.7	34.3	0	0	12.85	
Elk steak	168	3.2	34.7	0	0	10.84	
Venison roast	179	3.6	34.3	0	0	9.53	
Venison steak	179	3.6	34.3	0	0	9.53	
Bison top round steak	138	2.8	26.4	0	0	9.43	
Rabbit meat	196	4.0	37.4	0	0	9.35	
Elk loin	189	4.4	35.0	0	0	7.95	
Bison chuck shoulder	219	6.0	38.3	0	0	6.38	
Venison heart	187	5.4	32.3	0.17	0	5.80	Vitamin B12, potassium, selenium, and collagen
Bison rib-eye	200	6.4	33.4	0	0	5.22	
Bison top sirloin	194	6.4	31.8	0	0	4.97	
Venison liver	196	8.0	28.0	0	0	3.50	Almost everything, especially vitamins A, C, and D, folate, and minerals like magnesium, selenium, potassium, and zinc
Venison, ground	212	9.3	30.0	0	0	3.23	
Elk, ground	219	9.9	30.2	0	0	3.05	
Bison, ground	166	8.2	23.0	0	0	2.80	
Bison liver	241	5.3	33.3	6.7	0	2.78	Almost everything, especially vitamins A, C, and D, folate, and minerals like magnesium, selenium, potassium, and zinc
Bear meat	186	9.4	22.8	0	0	2.43	
Bison heart	239	16.0	22.7	0	0	1.42	Vitamin B12, potassium, selenium, and collagen

Venison refers specifically to deer in this case.

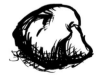

EGGS AND DAIRY (PER OUNCE UNLESS NOTED)	Calories	Fat	Protein	Carbs	Fiber	P/E ratio	Nutrients
Egg white (1 large)	17.4	0.06	3.64	0.24	0	12.13	
Plain Greek yogurt (0% fat, per cup)*	144.6	0.96	25.0	9.0	0	2.51	
Cottage cheese (4% fat)*	206	9	23.35	7.1	0	1.45	
Parmesan	111	7.32	10.13	0.91	0	1.23	
Plain Greek yogurt (whole milk, per cup)*	230	11.0	22.0	9.0	0	1.10	
Egg (1 large)	68.2	4.7	5.5	0.5	0.0	1.07	
Romano	109.7	7.64	9.0	1.03	0	1.04	
Mozzarella (part-skim)	83.6	5.61	6.73	1.58	0	0.94	
Gruyère	117	9.17	8.45	0.1	0	0.91	
Provolone	99.5	7.55	7.25	0.61	0	0.89	
Goat cheese	74.8	6.0	5.25	0	0	0.88	
Gouda	101	7.78	7.07	0.63	0	0.84	
Swiss	82.5	6.51	5.66	0.3	0	0.83	
Mozzarella (whole milk)	90	7.0	6.12	0.7	0	0.79	
Brie	94.7	7.85	5.88	0.13	0	0.74	
Ricotta (whole milk)	49.3	3.68	3.19	0.86	0	0.70	
Blue	100	8.15	6.07	0.66	0	0.69	
Gorgonzola	100	8.15	6.1	0.66	0	0.69	
Cheddar	114	9.44	6.48	0	0	0.69	
Stilton	116	9.9	6.72	0.03	0	0.68	
Roquefort	104.6	8.7	6.1	0.57	0	0.66	
Asiago	130	11.0	7.0	0.94	0	0.59	
Feta	74.8	6.0	4.0	1.16	0	0.56	
Egg yolk (1 large)	47	3.87	2.32	0.52	0	0.53	
Cream cheese	99	9.76	1.74	1.56	0	0.15	
Sour cream	28.5	2.78	0.35	0.67	0	0.10	
Mascarpone	121	12.83	0.95	1.12	0	0.07	
Butter	203	23.0	0.24	0.02	0	0.01	
Ghee	248	28.2	0.08	0	0	0.00	

*These products are higher in carbs, so you should limit or avoid them for best results.

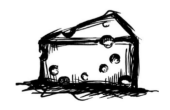

Butcher Charts

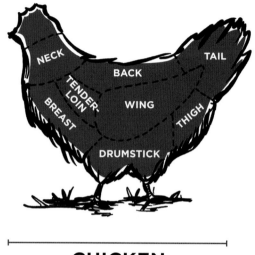

CHICKEN

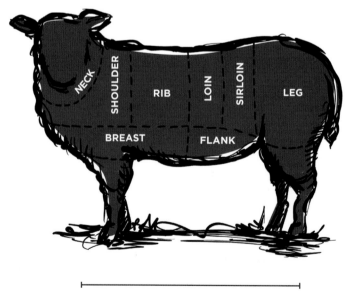

LAMB

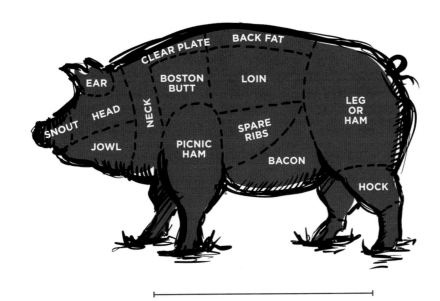

PORK

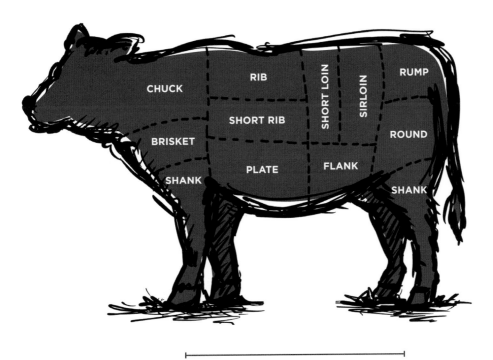

BEEF

Meat Temperature Guide

Blue, Pittsburgh
115°F (46°C)
Dark purple, cool, stringy, slippery, slightly juicy

RARE
125°F (52°C)
Bright purple-red center, warm, tender, juicy

MEDIUM RARE
CHEF TEMP: 135°F (57°C)
Bright red center, warm, tender, very juicy

MEDIUM
145°F (63°C)
Rich pink center, yielding, juicy

MEDIUM WELL
150°F (66°C)
Tan with slight pink, firm, slightly fibrous, slightly juicy

WELL DONE
160°F (71°C) or more
Tan to brown, no pink, chewy, dry

Lamb, venison, duck (steaks, chops, roasts)	**Medium Rare 130–135°F (54–57°C)** *USDA Min. 145°F (63°C)*	Bright red center, warm, tender, very juicy
Pork, fresh hams, veal (steaks, chops, roasts)	**Medium 135–145°F (57–63°C)** *USDA Min. 145°F (63°C)*	Cream-colored center, some pink, yielding, juicy
Pork ribs, pork shoulders, beef briskets, beef ribs	**190–205°F (88–96°C)** *USDA Min. 145°F (63°C)*	High in fat and collagen, best cooked low and slow
Chicken, turkey, including stuffing (whole or ground)	**160°F (71°C)** *USDA Min. 165°F (74°C)*	Cream-colored white meat, pale tan dark meat
Ground meats, burgers, sausages (precooked only)	**160°F (71°C)** *USDA Min. 160°F (71°C)*	Cook these risky meats to USDA minimum
Hams, hot dogs, sausages (precooked only)	**140°F (60°C) or more** *USDA Min. 140°F (60°C)*	Tender and juicy
Fish (except tuna steaks)	**Medium 130–145°F (54–63°C)** *USDA Min. 145°F (63°C)*	Slightly translucent, flaky, tender
Tuna steaks	**Rare 120–125°F (49–52°C)** *USDA Min. 145°F (63°C)*	Bright red center
Shrimp, lobster, crabs, scallops		Until flesh is opaque

USDA Grades of Beef

	MODERATELY ABUNDANT MARBLING	MODERATE MARBLING	SLIGHT MARBLING

MARBLING

The amount of fat streaking within the cut of meat

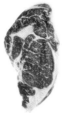 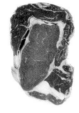 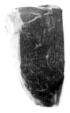

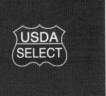

USDA PRIME BEEF

Produced from young, well-fed beef cattle. It has slightly abundant to abundant marbling and is generally sold in hotels and restaurants. Prime roasts and steaks are excellent for broiling, roasting, or grilling.

USDA CHOICE BEEF

High-quality but with less marbling than Prime. Choice roasts and steaks from the loin and rib are very tender, juicy, and flavorful and are suited for broiling, roasting, or grilling. Less tender cuts, such as from the round, are perfect for braising, roasting, or simmering on the stove with a small amount of liquid.

USDA SELECT BEEF

Normally leaner than Prime or Choice. It's fairly tender but it has less marbling, so it may not have as much juiciness or flavor. Select beef can be great on the grill, and it's also good for marinating or braising.

REFERENCES

Introduction

K. Beckman. "9 Factors That Affect Longevity." *ThinkAdvisor* website. May 27, 2016. Accessed at https://www.thinkadvisor.com/2016/05/27/9-factors-that-affect-longevity/?slreturn=20190506183852

Chapter 2

M. Angell. "Drug Companies & Doctors: A Story of Corruption." *The New York Review of Books* magazine. January 15, 2009. Accessed at https://www.nybooks.com/articles/2009/01/15/drug-companies-doctorsa-story-of-corruption/

G. Lundberg. "It's Not the Fat that Makes Us Unhealthy." *Medscape* video. August 24, 2018. Accessed at https://www.medscape.com/viewarticle/900495

V. Stefansson. *Cancer: Disease of Civilization? Anthropological and Historical Study* (New York: Hill and Wang, 1960).

Chapter 3

R. Aykroyd, D. Lucy, M. Pollard, and C. Roberts. "Nasty, Brutish, but Not Necessarily Short: A Reconsideration of the Statistical Methods Used to Calculate Age at Death from Adult Human Skeletal and Dental Age Indicators." *American Antiquity* 65, no. 1 (1999): 55–70.

D. Beasley, A. Koltz, J. Lambert, N. Fierer, and R. Dunn. "The Evolution of Stomach Acidity and Its Relevance to the Human Microbiome." *PLOS ONE* 10, no. 7 (2015).

California Academy of Sciences. "Oldest Evidence of Stone Tool Use and Meat-Eating Among Human Ancestors Discovered: Lucy's Species Butchered Meat." *Science Daily* website, August 11, 2010. Accessed at https://www.sciencedaily.com/releases/2010/08/100811135039.htm

D. Fisher. "Taphonomic Analysis of Late Pleistocene Mastodon Occurrences: Evidence of Butchery by North American Paleo-Indians." *Paleobiology* 10, no. 3 (1984): 338–57.

J. Hagelaars. "The Two Epochs of Marcott." *My View on Climate* blog. Accessed at https://ourchangingclimate.wordpress.com/2013/03/19/the-two-epochs-of-marcott/

J. Kuhn. "Throwing, the Shoulder, and Human Evolution." *American Journal of Orthopedics* 45, no. 2 (2016): 110–4.

C. Larsen. "Biological Changes in Human Populations with Agriculture." *Annual Review of Anthropology* 24, no. 1 (1995): 185–213.

Y. Malhi, C. Doughty, M. Galetti, F. Smith, J. Svenning, and J. Terborgh. "Megafauna and Ecosystem Function from the Pleistocene to the Anthropocene." *Proceedings of the National Academy of Sciences of the United States of America* 113, no. 4 (2016): 838–46.

K. Milton. "Nutritional Characteristics of Wild Primate Foods: Do the Diets of Our Closest Living Relatives Have Lessons for Us?" *Nutrition* 15, no. 6 (1999): 488–98.

C. Organ, C. Nunn, Z. Machanda, and R. Wrangham. "Phylogenetic Rate Shifts in Feeding Time During the Evolution of *Homo*." *Proceedings of the National Academy of Sciences of the United States of America* 108, no. 35 (2011): 14555–9.

B. Pobiner. "New Actualistic Data on the Ecology and Energetics of Hominin Scavenging Opportunities." *Journal of Human Evolution* 80 (2015): 1–16.

E. Trinkaus, A. Soficaru, A. Doboș, S. Constantin, J. Zilhão, and M. Richards. "Stable Isotope for Early Modern Human Diet in Southeastern Europe." *Academia* website. Accessed at http://www.academia.edu/245715/Stable_Isotope_Evidence_for_Early_Modern_Human_Diet_in_Southeastern_Europe_Pe%C5%9Ftera_cu_Oase_Pe%C5%9Ftera_Muierii_and_Pe%C5%9Ftera_Cioclovina_Uscat%C4%83

W. Zuo, F. Smith, and E. Charnov. "A Life-History Approach to the Late Pleistocene Megafaunal Extinction." *The American Naturalist* 182, no. 4 (2013): 524–31.

Chapter 4

P. Appleby, F. Crowe, K. Bradbury, R. Travis, and T. Key. "Mortality in Vegetarians and Comparable Nonvegetarians in the United Kingdom." *The American Journal of Clinical Nutrition* 103, no. 1 (2016): 218–30.

W. L. Braddon and E. A. Cooper. "The Influence of Metabolic Factors in Beri-Beri. Part I. The Effect of Increasing the Carbohydrate Ration on the Development of Polyneuritis in Birds Fed on Polished Rice." *The Journal of Hygiene* 14, no. 3 (1914): 331–53.

N. R. Cook et al. "A Randomized Factorial Trial of Vitamins C and E and Beta Carotene in the Secondary Prevention of Cardiovascular Events in Women: Results from the Women's Antioxidant Cardiovascular Study." *Archives of Internet Medicine* 167, no. 15 (2007): 1610–8.

M. Devries, A. Sithamparapillai, S. Brimble, L. Banfield, R. Morton, and S. Phillips. "Changes in Kidney Function Do Not Differ Between Healthy Adults Consuming Higher- Compared with Lower- or Normal-Protein Diets: A Systematic Review and Meta-Analysis." *The Journal of Nutrition* 148, no. 11 (2018): 1760–75.

D. Feldman. *Diet Doctor* website. Accessed at https://www.dietdoctor.com/authors/dave-feldman

D. Garfinkel and L. Garfinkel. "Magnesium and Regulation of Carbohydrate Metabolism at the Molecular Level." *Magnesium* 7, no. 5–6 (1988): 249–61.

J. Geraci and T. Smith. "Vitamin C in the Diet of Inuit Hunters from Holman, Northwest Territories." *Arctic* 32, no. 2 (1979): 135–8.

R. Ghodsi and S. Kheirouri. "Carnosine and Advanced Glycation End Products: A Systematic Review." *Amino Acids* 50, no. 9 (2018): 1177–86.

K. Ho, C. Tan, M. Daud, and F. Seow-Choen. "Stopping or Reducing Dietary Fiber Intake Reduces Constipation and Its Associated Symptoms." *World Journal of Gastroenterology* 18, no. 33 (2012): 4593–96.

S. J. Hur, C. Jo, Y. Yoon, and K. T. Lee. "Controversy on the Correlation of Red and Processed Meat Consumption with Colorectal Cancer Risk: An Asian Perspective." *Critical Reviews in Food Science and Nutrition* (2018): 1–12.

J. Jamnik et al. "Fructose Intake and Risk of Gout and Hyperuricemia: A Systematic Review and Meta-Analysis of Prospective Cohort Studies." *BMJ Open* 6 (2016): e013191.

S. Jarrett, J. Milder, L. Liang, and M. Patel. "The Ketogenic Diet Increases Mitochondrial Glutathione Levels." *Journal of Neurochemistry* 106, no. 3 (2008): 1044–51.

M. Kasielski, M. Eusebio, M. Pietruczuk, and D. Nowak. "The Relationship Between Peripheral Blood Mononuclear Cells Telomere Length and Diet: Unexpected Effect of Red Meat." *Nutrition Journal* 15, no. 1 (2016): 68.

D. Klurfeld. "What Is the Role of Meat in a Healthy Diet?" *Animal Frontiers* 8, no. 3 (2018): 5–10.

M. M. Mielke et al. "The 32-Year Relationship Between Cholesterol and Dementia from Midlife to Late Life." *Neurology* 75, no. 21 (2010): 1888–95.

T. Neogi, C. Chen, J. Niu, C. Chaisson, D. Hunter, and Y. Zhang. "Alcohol Quantity and Type on Risk of Recurrent Gout Attacks: An Internet-Based Case-Crossover Study." *The American Journal of Medicine* 127, no. 4 (2014): 311–8.

G. Parnaud, G. Peiffer, S. Taché, and D. E. Corpet. "Effect of Meat (Beef, Chicken, and Bacon) on Rat Colon Carcinogenesis." *Nutrition and Cancer* 32, no. 3 (1998): 165–73.

A. Peery et al. "A High-Fiber Diet Does Not Protect Against Symptomatic Diverticulosis." *Gastroenterology* 142, no. 2 (2012): 266–72.e1.

I. Schatz, K. Masaki, K. Yano, R. Chen, B. Rodriguez, and D. Curb. "Cholesterol and All-Cause Mortality in Elderly People from the Honolulu Heart Program: A Cohort Study." *The Lancet* 358, no. 9279 (2001): 351–55.

M. Sheffer and C. L. Taylor. *The Development of DRIs, 1994–2004: Lessons Learned and New Challenges Workshop Summary* (Washington, DC: The National Academies Press, 2008).

E. Sijbrands, R. Westendorp, J. Defesche, P. de Meier, A. Smelt, and J. Kastelein. "Mortality over Two Centuries in Large Pedigree with Familial Hypercholesterolaemia: Family Tree Mortality Study." *The BMJ* 322 (2001): 1019.

R. Sirtoli. "The Ultimate Keto Diet Guide for Beginners." *Nutrita* website. Updated May 27, 2019. Accessed at https://nutrita.app/complete-guide-to-ketogenic-diet-for-beginners/

F. Stirpe and M. Comporti. "Adaptive Regulation of Ascorbic Acid Synthesis in Rat-Liver Extracts. Effect of X-Irradiation and of Dietary Changes." *The Biochemical Journal* 86, no. 2 (1963): 232–6.

G. E. Thottam, S. Krasnokutsky, and M. H. Pillinger. "Gout and Metabolic Syndrome: A Tangled Web." *Current Rheumatology Reports* 19, no. 10 (2017): 60.

M. E. Van Elswyk, C. A. Weatherford, and S. H. McNeill. "A Systematic Review of Renal Health in Healthy Individuals Associated with Protein Intake Above the US Recommended Daily Allowance in Randomized Controlled Trials and Observational Studies." *Advances in Nutrition* 9, no. 4 (2018): 404–18.

A. Weverling-Rijnsburger, G. Blauw, M. Lagaay, D. Knock, E. Meinders, and R. Westendorp. "Total Cholesterol and Risk of Mortality in the Oldest Old." *The Lancet* 350, no. 9085 (1997): 1119–23.

G. Wu et al. "Proline and Hydroxyproline Metabolism: Implications for Animal and Human Nutrition." *Amino Acids* 40, no. 4 (2011): 1053–63.

C. S. Yajnik, R. F. Smith, T. D. Hockaday, and N. I. Ward. "Fasting Plasma Magnesium Concentrations and Glucose Disposal in Diabetes." *The BMJ* 288 (1984): 1032.

Chapter 5

G. Cavallini, S. Caracciolo, G. Vitali, F. Modenini, and G. Biagiotti. "Carnitine Versus Androgen Administration in the Treatment of Sexual Dysfunction, Depressed Mood, and Fatigue Associated with Male Aging." *Urology* 63, no. 4 (2004): 641–6.

A. R. Hipkiss. "Could Carnosine or Related Structures Suppress Alzheimer's Disease?" *Journal of Alzheimer's Disease* 11, no. 2 (2007): 229–40.

T. Huc et al. "Chronic, Low-Dose TMAO Treatment Reduces Diastolic Dysfunction and Heart Fibrosis in Hypertensive Rats." *Heart and Circulatory Physiology* 315, no. 6 (2018): H1805–20.

K. Mahajani and V. Bhatnagar. "Comparative Study of Prevalence of Anaemia in Vegetarian and Non Vegetarian Women of Udaipur City, Rajasthan." *Journal of Nutrition & Food Sciences* S3 (2015).

R. Mynatt. "Carnitine and Type 2 Diabetes." *Diabetes/Metabolism Research and Reviews* 25, supplement 1 (2009): S45–9.

R. Pawlak, S. J. Parrott, S. Raj, D. Cullum-Dugan, and D. Lucas. "How Prevalent Is Vitamin B12 Deficiency Among Vegetarians." *Nutrition Reviews* 71, no. 2 (2013): 110–17.

V. Senthong et al. "Intestinal Microbiota-Generated Metabolite Trimethylamine-*N*-Oxide and 5-Year Mortality Risk in Stable Coronary Artery Disease: The Contributory Role of Intestinal Microbiota in a COURAGE-Like Patient Cohort." *The Journal of the American Heart Association* 5, no. 6 (2016): e002816.

R. Smith, A. Agharkar, and E. Gonzales. "A Review of Creatine Supplementation in Age-Related Diseases: More than a Supplement for Athletes." *F1000Research* 3, no. 222 (2014). https://www.ncbi.nlm.nih.gov/pmc/articles/PMC4304302/

M. Soinio, J. Marniemi, M. Laakso, K. Pyörälä, S. Lehto, and T. Rönnemaa. "Serum Zinc Level and Coronary Heart Disease Events in Patients with Type 2 Diabetes." *DiabetesCare* 30, no. 3 (2007): 523–8.

C. G. Zhang and S. J. Kim. "Taurine Induces Anti-Anxiety by Activating Strychnine-Sensitive Glycine Receptor in vivo." *Annals of Nutrition & Metabolism* 51, no. 4 (2007): 379–86.

Chapter 6

B. N. Ames, M. Profet, and L. S. Gold. "Dietary Pesticides (99.99% All Natural)." *Proceedings of the National Academy of Sciences of the United States of America* 87, no. 19 (1990): 7777–81.

M. Bernardino and M. Parmar. "Oxalate Nephropathy from Cashew Nut Intake." *Canadian Medical Association Journal* 189, no. 10 (2017): E405–08.

I. F. Bolarinwa, M. O. Oke, S. A. Olaniyan, and A. S. Ajala. "A Review of Cyanogenic Glycosides in Edible Plants," chap. 8 in *Toxicology—New Aspects to This Scientific Conundrum* (Rijeka, Croatia: InTech, 2016).

S. Bugel, J. Bonventre, and R. Tanguay. "Comparative Developmental Toxicity of Flavonoids Using an Integrative Zebrafish System." *Toxicological Sciences* 154, no. 1 (2016): 55–68.

N. T. Davies. "Effects of Phytic Acid on Mineral Availability," in *Dietary Fiber in Health and Disease* (New York: Plenum Press, 1982), 105–16.

G. Ede. "Vegetables." *Diagnosis: Diet* website. Accessed at http://www.diagnosisdiet.com/food/vegetables/

J. M. Gee et al. "Effects of Saponins and Glycoalkaloids on the Permeability and Viability of Mammalian Intestinal Cells and on the Integrity of Tissue Preparations in Vitro." *Toxicology in Vitro* 10, no. 2 (1996): 117–28.

G. S. Gilani, C. W. Xiao, and K. Cockell. "Impact of Antinutritional Factors in Food Proteins on the Digestibility of Protein and the Bioavailability of Amino Acids and on Protein Quality." *British Journal of Nutrition* 108, no. 52 (2012): S315–32.

T. Gong et al. "Plant Lectins Activate the NLRP3 Inflammasome to Promote Inflammatory Disorders." *The Journal of Immunology* 198, no. 5 (2017): 2082–92.

S. Gundry. *The Plant Paradox: The Hidden Dangers in "Healthy" Foods That Cause Disease and Weight Gain* (New York: HarperCollins, 2017).

E. Lorenz, C. Michet, D. Milliner, and J. Lieske. "Update on Oxalate Crystal Disease." *Current Rheumatology Reports* 15, no. 7 (2013): 340.

S. Malakar. "Bioactive Food Chemicals and Gastrointestinal Symptoms: A Focus of Salicylates." *Journal of Gastroenterology and Hepatology* 32, no. 51 (2017): 73–7.

B. Patel, R. Schutte, P. Sporns, J. Doyle, L. Jewel, and R. N. Fedorak. "Potato Glycoalkaloids Adversely Affect Intestinal Permeability and Aggravate Inflammatory Bowel Disease." *Inflammatory Bowel Diseases* 8, no. 5 (2002): 340–6.

T. Truong, D. Baron-Dubourdieu, Y. Rougier, and P. Guénel. "Role of Dietary Iodine and Cruciferous Vegetables in Thyroid Cancer: A Countrywide Case-Control Study in New Caledonia." *Cancer Causes Control* 21, no. 8 (2010): 1183–92.

Chapter 7

J. Antonio, C. Peacock, A. Ellerbroek, B. Fromhoff, and T. Silver. "The Effects of Consuming a High Protein Diet (4.4 g/kg/d) on Body Composition in Resistance-Trained Individuals." *Journal of the International Society of Sports Nutrition* 11, no. 19 (2014): eCollection 2014.

N. Avena, P. Rada, and B. Hoebel. "Evidence for Sugar Addiction: Behavioral and Neurochemical Effects of Intermittent, Excessive Sugar Intake." *Neuroscience & Behavioral Reviews* 32, no. 1 (2008): 20–39.

S. Baker and M. Maier. *Track-Well Forum*. Updated June 6, 2018. Accessed at https://forum.track-well.com/t/carnivore-challenge-preliminary-results-are-good-weight-down-waist-down-pulse-down/42

A. Fasano. "Leaky Gut and Autoimmune Diseases." *Clinical Reviews in Allergy & Immunology.* 42, no. 1 (2012): 71–8.

W. Chai et al. "Dietary Red and Processed Meat Intake and Markers of Adiposity and Inflammation: The Multiethnic Cohort Study." *The Journal of the American College of Nutrition* 36, no. 5 (2017): 378–85.

R. Marshall. *Arctic Village.* Fairbanks, Alaska: University of Alaska Press, 1991.

F. Meader and E. Meader. *Year of the Caribou*, 1974, Alaska Wilderness Films.

C. Nasca et al. "Acetyl-L-Carnitine Deficiency in Patients with Major Depressive Disorder." *Proceedings of the National Academy of Sciences of the United States of America* 115, no. 34 (2018): 8627–32.

Paleomedicina website. Accessed at https://www.paleomedicina.com/en/#rolunk

L. Strath et al. "The Effect of Low-Carbohydrate and Low-Fat Diets on Pain in Individuals with Knee Osteoarthritis." *Pain Medicine* pnz022 (2019).

Chapter 8

C. Ebbeling et al. "Effects of a Low Carbohydrate Diet on Energy Expenditure During Weight Loss Maintenance: Randomized Trial." *The BMJ* 363, no. 8177 (2018): k4583.

M. A. Farhangi, S. Keshavarz, M. Eshraghian, A. Ostadrahimi, and A. Saboor-Yaraghi. "White Blood Cell Count in Women: Relation to Inflammatory Biomarkers, Haematological Profiles, Visceral Adiposity, and Other Cardiovascular Risk Factors." *Journal of Health, Population, and Nutrition* 31, no. 1 (2013): 58–64.

M. Den Heijer, S. Lewington, and R. Clarke. "Homocysteine, MTHFR and Risk of Venous Thrombosis: A Meta-Analysis of Published Epidemiological Studies." *Journal of Thrombosis and Haemostasis* 3, no. 2 (2005): 292–9.

D. Feldman. *Cholesterol Code* website. Accessed at https://cholesterolcode.com/

S. Gill and S. Panda. "A Smartphone App Reveals Erratic Diurnal Eating Patterns in Humans That Can Be Modulated for Health Benefits." *Cell Metabolism* 22, no. 5 (2015): 789–98.

L. A. Gilmore et al. "Consumption of High-Oleic Acid Ground Beef Increases HDL-Cholesterol Concentration but Both High- and Low-Oleic Acid Ground Beef Decrease HDL Particle Diameter in Normocholesterolemic Men." *The Journal of Nutrition* 141, no. 6 (2011): 1188–94.

E. Hopkins and S. Sharma. *Physiology, Acid Base Balance* (Treasure Island, FL: StatPearls Publishing, 2019). Accessed at https://www.ncbi.nlm.nih.gov/books/NBK507807/

S. Kashyap et al. "Ileal Digestibility of Intrinsically Labeled Hen's Egg and Meat Protein Determined with the Dual Stable Isotope Tracer Method in Indian Adults." *The American Journal of Clinical Nutrition* 108, no. 5 (2018): 980–7.

H. Kim, S. Lee, and R. Choue. "Metabolic Responses to High Protein Diet in Korean Elite Body Builders with High-Intensity Resistance Exercise." *Journal of the International Society of Sports Nutrition* 8 (2011): 10.

M. Safieh, A. Korczyn, and D. Michaelson. "ApoE4: An Emerging Therapeutic Target for Alzheimer's Disease." *BMC Medicine* 17, no. 64 (2019): 64.

S. Smith. "Marbling and Its Nutritional Impact on Risk Factors for Cardiovascular Disease." *Korean Journal for Food Science of Animal Resources* 36, no. 4 (2016): 435–44.

Chapter 10

K. Andersen and K. Kuhn. *Cowspiracy: The Sustainability Secret*, 2014, Appian Way.

J. Bentley. "U.S. Trends in Food Availability and a Dietary Assessment of Loss-Adjusted Food Availability, 1970–2014." *Economic Information Bulletin*, no. 166 (2017): 24.

M. Dehghan et al. "Associations of Fats and Carbohydrate Intake with Cardiovascular Disease and Mortality in 18 Countries from Five Continents (PURE): A Prospective Cohort Study." *The Lancet* 390, no. 10107 (2017): P2050–62.

B. Fischer and A. Lamey. "Field Deaths in Plant Architecture." *Journal of Agriculture and Environmental Ethics* 31, no. 4 (2018): 409–28.

A. Glatzle. "Questioning Key Conclusions of FAO Publications 'Livestock's Long Shadow' (2006) Appearing Again in 'Tackling Climate Change Through Livestock' (2013)." *Pastoralism: Research, Policy, and Practice* 4, no. 1 (2014).

Humane Research Council. "Study of Current and Former Vegetarians and Vegans," 2014. Accessed at https://faunalytics.org/wp-content/uploads/2015/06/Faunalytics_Current-Former-Vegetarians_Full-Report.pdf

Intergovernmental Panel on Climate Change. "2014 Synthesis Report." Accessed at https://ar5-syr.ipcc.ch/topic_summary.php

"Italian Beef Production Uses 25% Less Water." *Carni Sostenibili* website, March 22, 2016. Accessed at http://carnisostenibili.it/en/italian-beef-production-uses-25-less-water/

J. Johansen. "The Glass Walls Project." *AgWired* website, May 8, 2013. Accessed at http://agwired.com/2013/05/08/the-glass-walls-project/

T. Key, P. Appleby, E. Spencer, R. Travis, A. Roddam, and N. Allen. "Mortality in British Vegetarians: Results from the European Prospective Investigation into Cancer and Nutrition (EPIC-Oxford)." *The American Journal of Clinical Nutrition* 89, no. 5 (2009): 1613S–19S.

D. Layman. "Assessing the Role of Cattle in Sustainable Food Systems." *Nutrition Today* 53, no. 4 (2018): 160–5.

S. Mihrshahi, D. Ding, J. Gale, M. Allman-Farinelli, E. Banks, and A. E. Bauman. "Vegetarian Diet and All-Cause Mortality: Evidence from a Large Population-Based Australian Cohort–the 45 and Up Study." *Preventive Medicine* 97 (2017): 1–7.

M. Richter et al. "Vegan Diet. Position of the German Nutrition Society." *Ernährungs Umschau* 63, no. 4 (2016): 92–102.

H. Shibata, H. Nagai, H. Haga, S. Yasumura, T. Suzuki, and Y. Suyama. "Nutrition for the Japanese Elderly." *Nutrition and Health* 8, no. 2–3 (1992): 165–75.

M. Springmann et al. "Health-Motivated Taxes on Red and Processed Meat: A Modelling Study on Optimal Tax Levels and Associated Health Impacts." *PLOS ONE* (2018). Accessed at https://journals.plos.org/plosone/article?id=10.1371/journal.pone.0204139

H. Steinfeld. *Livestock's Long Shadow: Environmental Issues and Options* (Rome, Italy: Food and Agriculture Organization of the United Nations, 2006). Accessed at http://www.fao.org/3/a-a0701e.pdf

United States Environmental Protection Agency. "Inventory of U.S. Greenhouse Gas Emissions and Sinks." Accessed at https://www.epa.gov/ghgemissions/inventory-us-greenhouse-gas-emissions-and-sinks

D. Widmar. "Pass the Meat: U.S. Meat Consumption Turns Higher." *Agricultural Economic Insights* website, October 31, 2016. Accessed at http://ageconomists.com/2016/10/31/u-s-meat-consumption-turns-higher/

World Health Organization. "Depression in India: Let's Talk." 2017. Accessed at http://www.searo.who.int/india/depression_in_india.pdf

INDEX

Y

Z